IF YOU LIKE EXERCISE . . .
CHANCES ARE YOU'RE DOING IT
WRONG

IF YOU LIKE EXERCISE . . . CHANCES ARE YOU'RE DOING IT WRONG

PROPER STRENGTH TRAINING FOR MAXIMUM RESULTS

GARY BANNISTER

iUniverse, Inc.
Bloomington

If You Like Exercise . . . Chances Are You're Doing It Wrong
Proper Strength Training for Maximum Results

iUniverse books may be ordered through booksellers or by contacting:

iUniverse
1663 Liberty Drive
Bloomington, IN 47403
www.iuniverse.com
1-800-Authors (1-800-288-4677)

ISBN: 978-1-4759-7439-3 (sc)
ISBN: 978-1-4759-7441-6 (hc)
ISBN: 978-1-4759-7440-9 (ebk)

Library of Congress Control Number: 2013902857

Printed in the United States of America

iUniverse rev. date: 02/22/2013

CONTENTS

INDEX—CHARTS AND DIAGRAMS

ACKNOWLEDGEMENTS

My thesis advisor, Celeste Ulrich, Ph.D., University of North Carolina at Greensboro who encouraged my talent for writing and, so often, went beyond the call of duty.

Digby Sale, Ph.D., my exercise physiology professor at McMaster University (Hamilton, Ontario) whose enthusiasm cultivated an interest in his subject, and who first introduced me to a Nautilus® machine.

Michael N. Fulton, M.D., orthopedic representative for Nautilus Sports/Medical Industries and MedX Corporation, whose belief in exercise clearly raised the bar of what physicians can and should be, and whose friendship I cherish.

Jim Flanagan, General Manager of Nautilus Sports/Medical Industries and MedX Corporation, whose generosity and hospitality introduced me to the dynamic medical lectures of Arthur Jones.

Ellington Darden, Ph.D., whose writings formed a basis for the practical application of proper strength-training theory—inspiring thousands to train in a safe, sane manner.

Brian D. Johnston, IART founder and president, whose written works provided information and inspiration for much of the content.

"Mr. Nautilus" John Turner, a friend and fellow author whose knowledge and resources were helpful throughout.

Judy Barre, a longtime friend whose support, suggestions and reading skills were fundamental to the final product.

William E. Jones, son of Arthur Jones, who granted permission to quote from his father's work.

Arthur Jones, a master teacher who challenged everyone he met to "think." His impatient, intolerant facade often dissipated the moment you showed a genuine interest and he would NOT abandon an inquiry until it was clear that you understood IN FULL. A rare bird—truly missed.

DEDICATION

....

Nautilus® inventor, Arthur Jones spent a lifetime examining cause and effect, searching for "truth" at a time when the field of exercise showed little interest in the same. His journey was influenced by a statement made long before: *"Instead of trying to determine how much exercise we can tolerate, perhaps we should try to determine how little we actually require."*

Early on he pursued the "gurus" of his day—by letter, by phone, by knocking on doors—and was impressed with their welcome but not their answers. Jones was cocky, persistent and—more important—brilliant. He decided to go it alone, entering the commercial end of the field in 1970 to a cold reception: Few could grasp his approach and fewer tried. Arthur was a threat to an establishment not accustomed to "truth" and—as was his style—openly revealed his hand:

> *". . . the only rational reason for reading any of this is an attempt to learn something. If, however, they (readers) are merely looking for additional confirmation of firmly-held beliefs, then we would strongly advise them to skip the rest of our writing. Because careful research and simple logic have already taught us that most of the current beliefs on the subject of exercise are without basis in fact, and experience has taught us that many people are apparently unwilling to change their beliefs, regardless of the evidence that is presented . . . we also know that the entire field of exercise will remain firm in the presently existing dark ages until and unless the light of logic is turned on the subject."*

Jones was a logical thinker and possibly the first genius to apply his talents to the subject. His depth of thought was profound, his delivery bold and to the point, his information backed by intellect, logic and experience. Arthur had few friends he trusted and was intolerant of fools. I was fortunate to be among the "tolerated"—lectures, lunches, dinners and a few one-on-ones. He could make you comfortable but more often you were not—always on the edge of your seat, listening in awe and sweating as the moments passed.

He was intense, interesting, unique. At his passing I felt—like many others—that I owed him something. I wrote a tribute before his time was up—a lengthy book he refused to read and Arthur was a reader. My thought: *If it wasn't from the horse's mouth, it must be from the other end.*

So I'm back; his work, my words—dedicated to a generation yet exposed to what Arthur Jones believed was the plain and simple "truth."

INTRODUCTION

· ·

Mickey didn't need exercise. With a 21-inch neck, 73-inch chest and 25-inch arms, he could do one-arm chin-ups "'til the cows came home"—and never once touched a barbell.

No one knew his age, but everyone knew he was pampered. When I first saw him, communication was one-way. Mickey refused to acknowledge anyone and spent most days as would any male—watching TV with a remote. His choices: Soap operas and American football.

When I last saw him, Mickey was lifeless—a stuffed version of the Wal-Mart® greeter at the entrance to the Center for Exercise Science at the University of Florida. It was no laughing matter to his owner. According to some, the man who invented Nautilus® machines treated Mickey better than members of his own family.

Arthur Jones purchased the primate from a circus, which made Mickey the only African lowland gorilla in captivity in a private collection. And Jones knew animals—it was his business. He housed the beauty in a cage the exact size of that at the circus to make him feel "at home" and then built an addition to make the enclosure three to four times larger and L-shaped—the original space plus a glassed-in extension that formed the interior wall of a sixty-foot-thick concrete tunnel.

The tunnel connected the runway of the world's largest private jetport to a conference facility where Jones hosted daily seminars *"to educate medical doctors."* The jetport was nothing to sneeze at—a 747, three 707's, fourteen other airplanes and—on occasion—The Concorde®. Jones did things IN LARGE and animal care was no exception. The tunnel wall shielded his collection from the noise of the jets while the glass yielded a view of the beast before conference proceedings. But Mickey refused to cooperate. He would not enter the extension.

They lured him with bananas to no avail. The great ape reached for the bait but always kept a large toe in the cage. Call it what you will, Mickey refused to leave the comforts of home.

In many ways his behavior resembles the body's reluctance to change. Every time you exercise, the body is forced to adjust its physiology to accommodate the "intrusion," which is why frequent exercise attracts the same routine(s) and why trainers preach the same sermon despite their occasional rush to certify in the latest. Change is threat, and threat, according to Jones, elicits a sequential response: Ignore, ridicule, adopt, copy and steal.

I have been labeled as not "current" in the field of exercise. Others claim that I am reluctant to change, stuck in the past, beating a dead horse and not open-minded. I can see more than assumed but the more I click the remote, the worse the picture. For the past half-century the field of exercise has marched backwards: From a "thinking man's barbell" to no barbell at all, from full-range to partial-range exercise, from valid tools to toys, from great to poor—all in the name of "progress." Along the way someone declared that the muscles of the "core" were important, that traditional training with barbells and machines was "non-functional," that body weight was the preferred resistance, that balance and circus stunts were missing links to athletic performance, and finally, that there were enough dummies out there to plow it through. Jones put it his way, *"Not all people are idiots, but they follow the advice of idiots, usually in the form of self-proclaimed experts."*

Arthur Jones was the outspoken inventor of Nautilus® (and later, MedX®) exercise and rehabilitation machines. The significance of his contributions to the fields of exercise and rehabilitative medicine are beyond the scope of a single publication. In brief, he developed tools that improved the quality and application of resistance to working muscles and created a more efficient, effective method of attaining physical goals—the Nautilus system, aptly named "Proper Strength Training." His new tools and system changed exercise forever and changed it for the better.

Initial exposures to the innovative training ended as did mine. I was twenty-five at the time, a physical-education instructor and coach at Averett College in Danville, Virginia. I had lifted weights and ran long distance three times a week for eleven years, participated in a variety of sports and was bullet-proof. When a fellow professor invited me to a new Nautilus gym in town, I bit. The space wasn't large or elegant, but the equipment was. Ten big, blue muscle-machines lined the walls, but I'd never see them all that day. The owner, more obsessed with protein shakes than training, pushed me through a combination leg extension/leg press machine that was the size of my bedroom—the Compound Leg. He then directed me to *quickly* mount an adjacent prone Leg Curl machine. My legs buckled as they hit the floor but it bolstered my resolve. I survived the Leg Curl and was whisked to a Pullover machine that I had tried two years before at my Alma Mater. I began what Jones called his "upper-body squat" but didn't last long. After four repetitions it felt like someone had dipped a drinking straw into my skull. I was clammy, nauseated and breathing like a freight train, and promptly headed for the men's room where I spent the next ten minutes. I could NOT continue—was "wiped out" the rest of the day—and could NOT believe my inability to tolerate six minutes of exercise. It made me realize that there was something more.

If You Like Exercise . . . Chances Are You're Doing It Wrong exposes that "something more" by presenting the concepts of intensity, duration, frequency, form, speed of motion, number of repetitions and full-range exercise in a clear, logical manner (as they were in the Nautilus glory days), this time with support from current research. It will lead its audience down an efficient, effective path to physical superiority in a way that finally "makes sense." It also exposes the so-called "something more" offered by the current crop of self-proclaimed experts—nothing more than inferior training concepts.

"Quite frankly," said Jones during his heyday, *"most of the people involved in exercise disgusted me, and I clearly understood that a very large percentage of them were either fools or frauds, or both. A situation that has changed primarily in the direction of becoming more widespread."*

Astro-physicist, Carl Sagan expressed it his way: *"One of the saddest lessons in history is this: If we've been bamboozled long enough, we tend to reject any evidence of the bamboozle. We're no longer interested in finding out the truth. The bamboozle has captured us. It is simply too painful* to acknowledge—even to ourselves—that we've been so credulous. So the old bamboozles tend to persist as the new bamboozles rise."

Arthur printed Sagan's quote on poster board for his conference guests—too little too late. The field of exercise was "neck deep in outright fraud and foolishness" and Jones could not turn the tide, even though some thought he had. The man who set out "to reach a small part of humanity" ended up, in some way or another, influencing everyone who has exercised since. But truth did not prevail . . .

Max Planck, inventor of the quantum theory in physics in 1900 explained why: *"A new scientific discovery does not prevail by convincing its opponents and leading them to see the light, but only because its opponents will eventually die and then a new generation will grow up who are aware of the truth."* A slow process.

Like Mickey, no one knew Arthur's age. He had three stock responses, one of which was, *"I'm old enough to realize it's impossible to change the thinking of fools. But I'm young and foolish enough to keep on trying."* And try he did—dedicating every waking hour to the truth and conducting research around one principle, "Let the chips fall where they may." He invariably answered unsolved questions with, "Let's find out"—and then followed-up. In the end it was apparent that the field of exercise was not comfortable with the truth—big money could be made without it.

"I am arrogant enough to believe," said Jones in the end, *"that my lifetime of interest in the field of exercise has produced developments that can provide great benefits to millions of other people if my discoveries and developments are not flushed down the toilet of history."*

The medical community has a large and heavy hand on the crank. People will listen to the advice of a physician over that of a trainer who suggests the same, "You need exercise." Unfortunately, there are fewer doctors than trainers who understand the value of exercise, and fewer yet who are aware of—or believe in—the contributions of Arthur Jones to the fields of exercise and rehabilitative medicine. After all, he quit school in grade four.

"During the last thirty years," he said, *"most of the worthwhile characteristics of civilization, no small part of the Earth itself, and practically all of the benefits of progressive exercise have been so perverted that almost nothing of value remains; the problems are known, but ignored—the answers are available, but denied—primarily, it seems, because far too many people are interested only in avoiding controversy or are unwilling to face up to difficult solutions."*

To his followers it wasn't the outcome that mattered, it was the effort—and with Jones, the effort was always IN LARGE. According to Jim Bryan, Jones went *"FAR out of his way to help people,"* which is why reference to his ideas and accomplishments in this book is deliberate, frequent and necessary. Exercise physiology hasn't changed: The potential benefits of exercise can be obtained in a single package—Proper Strength Training.

At a time when most offerings in the field of exercise require a courtesy flush, the words of Arthur Jones resound, *"The truth cannot be ignored forever."*

PART I

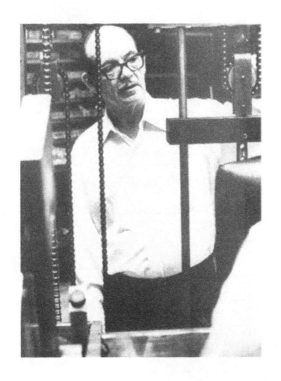

"We Now Know . . ."

CHAPTER 1

··

Intensity: The Cornerstone

I n mid-1968 Arthur Jones flew his family to Florida following a decade of work in the large-animal/film-making business in Africa. He was broke. All of his possessions had been confiscated by the Rhodesian government—but there was good news. He now had time to pursue a personal hobby—bodybuilding—and continue development of better tools for the purpose. He had abandoned several prototype machines in the jungle and had the latest seized.

Jones' training style was legendary. He kept meticulous records—every repetition, set, bodyweight, measurements—and decided to write about his progress by submitting an article to Bob Hoffman's *Strength and Health* magazine. No reply. He then sent it to Joe Weider's *Muscle Builder/Power* magazine. No reply. Frustrated, he reworked the piece into an attack on bodybuilding practices: *"Quit emulating the workouts of the men who are winning the titles,"* he wrote. *"Most of them can't even spell the word 'muscle.'"* His formula was simple but radical:

> *"If you want to get bigger and stronger, you must make measurable, stair-step progress during each workout. Size always precedes strength. If you're not making gains workout by workout, your exercise intensity is too low. The key is to train harder, to continue each exercise until no additional repetitions are possible. But if you train harder, you must train less."* [1]

Jones finally sent the article to Peary Rader's *Ironman* and was pleasantly surprised. Rader found it interesting and asked Arthur to write monthly articles for the magazine, which he did from 1970-74.

In 1973 Ellington Darden began writing for Jones' new entity, Nautilus Sports/ Medical Industries® and witnessed several of his workouts. Nearly a decade later, after training hundreds of world-class athletes in nearly every sport, he was asked, "Who trained the hardest?" His reply was swift, "Arthur Jones."

Due to his contributions to the field—and well after the fact—Jones became known as "The Father of High-Intensity Training." His hard-hitting system, "Proper Strength Training" (a fast-paced circuit of full-out exercise with little to no rest between efforts) evolved into "High-Intensity Training" or HIT, with advocates creating a global industry of literature, websites and trainer-certification organizations—a fitting tribute, but one that did not change perception.

To most, the phrases "High-Intensity Training" and "momentary muscle failure" evoke images of bodybuilders slamming massive weights in a chaotic mix of sweat and injury.

Both are mistakenly perceived as difficult and dangerous.

Difficult It Is

In *The Nautilus Bodybuilding Book* (1982), Ellington Darden described a workout he witnessed in Deland, Florida. The trainer was Arthur Jones; the trainees, Casey Viator (Mr. America, 1971) and the greatest threat to Schwarzenegger's dominance, Sergio Oliva:

"Casey began by performing 25 nonstop repetitions on a leg press machine with 460 pounds. Immediately he was hustled from the leg press to the leg extension where he did 22 repetitions with 200 pounds.

By now Viator's heart rate was in excess of 220 beats per minute, he was breathing like a steam engine, and sweat was pouring from his body. But there was no time to rest.

Instantly, Jones raced Casey to the squat rack where a barbell was loaded with 400 pounds. Then, Viator ground out 17 continuous repetitions in the full squat.

'Ok, Sergio, you're up,' said Jones, as Casey, unable to walk, slithered to the nearest hiding place.

Oliva reached the squat rack after 17 repetitions with 460 pounds in the leg press and 16 repetitions in the leg extension with 200 pounds. When Sergio broke the lock in his knees for the squat with 400 pounds, he went to the floor as if he had been knocked in the head. After being helped to his feet, he tried it again—with the same results. One hundred pounds were removed from the bar, during which delay Sergio was afforded some rest, and then he performed seven repetitions with 300 pounds.

Sergio was accustomed to training his legs for at least one hour almost nonstop in the traditional fashion. But during his leg workout under Jones' supervision, one cycle of three exercises performed until momentary muscular exhaustion within a period of five minutes was all he wanted. Furthermore, Sergio spent a considerably longer period of time stretched out in front of the gym.

When Sergio recovered sufficiently to continue his workout, the torso cycle and the arm cycle were completed in approximately 12 minutes. Previously, his torso and arm training had taken two hours or longer to complete.

But, obviously, Sergio Oliva had never trained with the intensity that he experienced with Jones and Viator.

Arnold Schwarzenegger also went through a similar training session under Jones' watchful eye and remarked, 'I've often experienced times during a workout where I had difficulty walking. But this is the first time that I've ever had difficulty lying down.'" [2]

Jones described his approach to training as "outright hard work." When all was said and done, few were left standing for the photo shoot. *"Cheese:"* he said, *"You can slice it as thin as you can, or pile it as high as you like—but you still end up with cheese. You can kid yourself any way you like—but you can't change facts; hard exercise—and ONLY HARD EXERCISE—produces worthwhile results in the way of muscular strength and size increases. If you are not willing to work hard, then FORGET IT—there simply isn't any other way to do it."* [3]

No explanation required.

I once asked a bodybuilder who entered my facility in Caracas, Venezuela for the first time what weight he could press overhead for ten repetitions. He replied, "Ciento veinte," (120 pounds). I needed to select a resistance for his effort on a Nautilus Double Shoulder machine which he had never used. The machine featured a lateral raise *and* overhead press exercise from a single seat. I cleaned the poor guy out on the lateral raise and quickly changed the weight for the press. He barely made the first repetition and struggled until he could lift no more. After a Spanish expletive, he asked, "Quanto?" (How much?). "Thirty pounds," I replied and escorted him to the rear of the machine to verify what he could not believe. He had nothing left after the first exercise. His effort was high but his output was low, as Jones explains:

"It should now be obvious that intensity is a relative situation depending upon momentary ability, varying moment by moment, and not directly related to output. If the trainee could have done more, but did not, then the intensity was low. But the intensity is maximum if he is doing all he can at the moment regardless of how much or how little output is actually involved." [4]

This guy did well to make five.

Dangerous It Is Not

Jones often called high-intensity exercise, "the safest way to train." Some found it hard to swallow.

Cheese: You can slice it as thin as you can, or pile it as high as you like—but you still end up with cheese. You can kid yourself any way you like—but you can't change facts; hard exercise—and ONLY HARD EXERCISE—produces worthwhile results in the way of muscular strength and size increases. If you are not willing to work hard, then FORGET IT—there simply isn't any other way to do it.

Danger exists—and injury occurs—when the force a muscle produces (or is exposed to) exceeds its structural integrity. Injury prevention requires strengthening muscles and/or exposing them to low force. Both are possible during high-intensity exercise, but let's first define terms.

Intensity is *a percentage of momentary ability.* Maximum intensity of contraction occurs when a muscle pulls with as much force as it can *momentarily* produce.

Intensity and resistance are independent. Resistance is *the weight used during exercise;* intensity, *the effort required to lift the weight.* It is possible and desirable to create a high level of intensity (effort) during exercise and keep forces produced by the effort low. In fact, it happens automatically during the performance of a set of repetitions, as described:

"Regardless of the number of repetitions involved in a set, the first repetition is ALWAYS the most dangerous repetition—and the last repetition is ALWAYS the safest repetition; and the harder it feels, the easier it is—and the more dangerous it appears, the safer it is.

The last repetition of a set of ten repetitions, for example, 'feels' harder only because you are becoming exhausted by that point in the set—you do not 'feel' actual output, instead you 'feel' the percentile of momentarily-possible output; if a man can press 200 pounds, then 100 pounds will 'feel light' to him during a first repetition, and will 'feel' heavier during each following repetition—and by the time he reaches a point where he is barely capable of performing one more repetition, then the 100 pounds will 'feel' very heavy. Because—to him, AT THAT MOMENT— 100 pounds actually will be very heavy, since it will momentarily require 100 percent of his strength to move it.

Everything is relative insofar as 'feelings' are concerned—a puma looks big to a man that has never seen a lion; but the danger of injury is not based on relative factors in that sense—instead, the connective tissues have an actual level of resistance to pull, and since they are not performing work this resistance is not reduced during the performance of a set of several repetitions. If a particular tendon's connective tissues have an existing level of resistance capable of withstanding 'one hundred units of pull,' then that level of resistance remains constant throughout the set—it will be one hundred units during the first repetition and 100 units during the tenth repetition; but the 'danger factor' certainly does NOT remain constant—because during a first repetition you might be momentarily capable of exerting 200 units of pull, and if you do then an injury literally MUST result, but by the time you reach the tenth repetition your momentary ability may be reduced to a maximum of only 10 units of pull, and you couldn't hurt yourself then if you tried, you simply are not strong enough to hurt yourself at that point." [5]

Fatigue is the key to safety and is built into every set of exercise . . . but only if you behave. Select a weight you can perform for (barely) ten repetitions in good form. During the first repetition, move more slowly than you are capable. At that juncture you *can* produce a force two-to-three times that of the resistance selected if you jerk the weight—not smart when the breaking strength of the involved tissues is unknown. During the second, third and fourth repetitions, the possibilities remain the same, but the danger has diminished repetition by repetition. At ten repetitions the involved muscle will have lost, on average, approximately 20% of its strength. A full effort at that point—involving a muscle that is capable of producing only 80% of its capacity—is much safer than the dynamics of the initial repetitions. Nonetheless, perform *all* repetitions (especially the first few) using a smooth, slow, controlled speed to reduce the chance of injury. Resist the temptation to jerk the weight.

Neurological Safety

Besides fatigue, the body has another built-in safety mechanism. During a 100% effort, only a small percentage of a muscle's available fibers become involved. An average muscle allows approximately 30% of its fibers to activate in an all-out, one-time lift. Some individuals, by birth, can recruit as much as 50% of their available fibers; others, only 10%. The 50-percenters are strong and powerful individuals; the 10-percenters, weaker by design. The fibers that are not activated lie in wait for future use or emergencies. The body MUST keep a reserve.

If a 50-percenter is forced to repeat a task, his 50% reserve will not last long—a few repetitions and out. In contrast, the 90% reserve of a 10-percenter comes in handy during repetitive tasks.

The maximum effort involved during high-intensity training does not change these values. The body will not allow a greater activation of fibers . . . for safety reasons. If and when ALL of a muscle is allowed to contract (such as during an electrocution or emergency—a loved one pinned under a car), bones break—something the body can do without.

Overload and Muscle Recruitment

The individual muscle fibers that are recruited during physical effort perform on an all-or-none basis—are either fully involved or not involved at all. The difficulty of the task dictates which fibers and how many are involved. When the task is easy, as it "feels" during the first repetitions of a set, only a few fibers are involved and are working as hard as they can. As the working fibers fatigue, the body judiciously taps the reserves to continue. The number of involved fibers changes from repetition to repetition. Terminating a set of exercise after only a few repetitions does nothing to stimulate change because of the large number of untapped muscle fibers. Stimulation most likely occurs when exercise is continued to a point where as many fibers as possible are involved, and where some of the fibers are worked to exhaustion.

A set of repetitions terminated prior to momentary muscle failure will not involve the maximum number of available fibers. Nor will it activate the powerful "fast-twitch" fibers which are recruited *only* when intensity is high. Both factors are crucial to stimulating growth, as Jones suggests: *"A slight decrease in the intensity of effort in exercise will result in a disproportionately great reduction in the production of results."* [6] He made the same clear to me one day with his finger in my face, *"Young man, if you perform ten repetitions of an exercise when you could have done twelve, you may as well stay in the parking lot. You'll get the same result—nothing."*

> **Fatigue, the key to safety, is built into every set of exercise . . . but only if you behave.**

The body loves to do nothing beyond its daily routine. To trigger a signal for change, muscles require: ONE, an overload—a resistance or challenge that exceeds the norm; and TWO, intensity—the involvement of a high percentage of momentary ability.

Practical Application

There are two ways to increase intensity during a workout: Work harder on each exercise performed and spend less time between efforts. Both come with a warning.

The 100% effort required at the moment your ability has been significantly reduced by fatigue is not something the body looks forward to. It doesn't like intrusion, much less an intense one—and there's proof. Trainees, left to their own, revert to "easier" habits that fail to satisfy the requirements for change. Effort must be all-out and **learned**. You can't show up one day determined to fail on every exercise because someone told you it was a good thing. Trainees must *gradually* increase effort until a complete repetition becomes impossible, which may take a while. Jones claimed that a highly motivated athlete armed with clear instructions concerning the necessary requirements might fail on one or two exercises (of twelve) when left to his own. In that regard and when possible, have your workouts supervised and pushed by a buddy or professional trainer.

In the initial stages of training rest after each exercise or you may find yourself staring at the lights. I'd rather see new trainees learn to work as hard as they can and rest for five minutes between efforts than do a little here and there. Gradually and with discretion, move quickly from one exercise to another, but be warned—the cost is high. Rapid movement between exercises demands chemical changes that initially can't be met. The resulting symptoms—lightheadedness, nausea, cold sweat and fainting—are signs that the pace is too quick. Don't be eager to get there. Time your total workout and *gradually* reduce it to a more efficient level. And don't be fooled: A twelve-exercise workout performed in seventeen minutes is **much more intense** than the same performed in twenty-five.

Arthur Jones likened muscle stimulation to tapping a stick of dynamite repeatedly with a hammer. Nothing happens. Now, take the hammer and SMASH it once—something happens. Intensity is the cornerstone of Proper Strength Training: It turns the switch "ON."

A slight decrease in the intensity of effort in exercise will result in a disproportionately great reduction in the production of results.

REFERENCES

[1] Darden, E., Ph.D., *The New High Intensity Training*, Rodale, Inc., 2: 13, 2004.

[2] Darden, E., Ph.D., *The Nautilus Bodybuilding Book*, Contemporary Books, 7: 50-51, 1982.

[3] Jones, A., *Nautilus Training Principles*, Bulletin No. 2, 18: 50, 1971. cheese

[4] Jones, A., "Progressive Exercise," Peterson, J.A., Ph.D. (editor), *Total Fitness the Nautilus Way*, Leisure Press, 4: 48, 1978.

[5] Jones, A., *Nautilus Training Principles*, Bulletin No. 2, 31: 89, 1971.

[6] Jones, A., *Nautilus Training Principles*, Bulletin No. 2, 30: 86, 1971.

CHAPTER 2

··

Proper Strength Training

"Steady-state (aerobic) training is necessary for cardiovascular benefits and non steady-state exercise (progressive resistance) is required for meaningful strength increases. Both results can be produced from the same training program."

Arthur Jones

M y first exposure to Proper Strength Training occurred in Virginia in 1973. It was followed years later by a glimpse of its commercial application near the University of Florida. The Gainesville Health and Fitness Center was a showcase of Nautilus equipment from day one. I was greeted by a sea of machines when I arrived, many of which were duplicates. There's nothing more impressive than ten to twelve identical tools in a line—line after line. But the effect was as functional as aesthetic. Each line represented a unique sequence supervised by trainers wearing shirt and tie.

The scene was deceptive. The "Yes, Sirs" and "No, Sirs" were soon overshadowed by forceful, motivating commands that left trainees barely in shorts by the end. The place bustled with energy and something less apparent—peer pressure. Trainees felt obligated to retain their position in the firing line, at times not easy. The workout for those who made it was worthy of note.

I modeled my facility in Caracas around what I saw that day. Twelve machines, and later twenty-five, were barely a "sea"—and the shirt-and-tie challenge a bit too much—but I devised a method that preserved the integrity of the system. Every client was "supervised and pushed" during every workout for ten years . . . and I learned a few things along the way:

- Proper Strength Training was effective. Most clients made significant gains and when results did not match expectations, lack of form or intensity was generally at fault.
- It was efficient. Thirty minutes or less, three times a week at most, was not a large investment in time.
- And it was enough. When clients were "pushed" (relative to their condition) on a clear runway, the program was all they could handle.

What was done? We encouraged trainees to work as hard as they could (eventually to a point of momentary muscle failure) on each exercise and move as quickly as they could to the next—the essence of Proper Strength Training.

It wasn't always that way.

It started, in fact, with three four-hour workouts per week, four sets of exercise and not much rest between. The man at the end of the barbell was not what you would call "patient." He demanded results from *every* repetition, *every* set, *every* workout—but it didn't happen. His arms and calves grew quickly, while other parts lagged. Frustration set in and he quit—a good thing, because the man at the end of the barbell was a thinker. Months, often years, passed before he returned with a new plan . . . but the result was always the same.

He attacked the equipment. The "miracle tool" he so often used had failed his lagging torso muscles—did not provide direct exercise or adequate resistance to those muscles when they reached a position of full contraction, a simple FACT of barbell training.

All free-weight exercises designed to stimulate growth in the large muscles of the torso are indirect: The upper arms are the venue of access. Chest and shoulder exercises, for example, involve triceps; upper-back exercises, biceps. In all cases and because of relative size, the muscles of the upper-arm (and sometimes the forearm) fatigue *before* the muscles of the torso, which limits the possibility of their stimulation and explains our thinker's description of his results, *"the arms of a gorilla on the body of a spider monkey."* But he wasn't done. Movement of the upper-arm triggers movement of the upper-back, chest and shoulder muscles. The application of pads to the upper-arm would transfer resistance directly to those muscles and any effort against the pad would fatigue large rather than small muscles—"a thinking man's barbell."

Free-weights did not "feel" right for another reason. The frustration of biceps curls forced him to weld a chain to each end of the barbell. When his forearms passed the mid-point of their effort (when they were parallel to the floor), the chains sequentially lifted added resistance from the floor to make the full-contracted position "feel" heavier—which established the need to deliver a variable resistance to the muscle as it moved through its range of motion.

But that wasn't enough. In most cases, available muscle strength increases as movement approaches contraction and then decreases. The impracticality of welded chains spawned the birth of the exercise "cam" and all the innovations that followed.

At the same time he examined his training system and left no stone unturned. He changed every parameter—speed of movement, exercise sequence and choice, number of repetitions and time parameters—in an effort to increase results. Every attempt led to the same dead end. At 5'8", he reached but could not surpass a bodyweight of 172 pounds. One day he decided to perform *less* exercise, two sets instead of four. By week's end and with no other modifications, he gained ten pounds and couldn't believe it. Work forced him to quit for a year. When he returned, he continued to *decrease* the amount of exercise performed and "peaked" at a solid 205 pounds with a cold-arm measurement of 17¼ inches. *"It took me twenty years to discover that two sets of exercise were better than four,"* he declared, *"and another ten to discover that one set was better than two."*

It was time to share his discovery.

With new tools and a fledgling philosophy in hand, Arthur Jones invited anyone to train under his guidance in Lake Helen, Florida, 1970. The free offer was no bargain. Of the many that showed, some vowed *never* to return; others believed—as they lay sprawled on the floor—that he was "on to something."

That same year he invited a young man who had placed tenth in the Mr. America contest to work for him and train under his guidance. The next year, Casey Viator won the event in spectacular fashion, capturing "best" in every category (except abdomen) and youngest ever (at age nineteen). The results sent shock-waves through the bodybuilding community.

Word got out: The new method worked but was "Hell on rubbery legs." No one but Viator could do it. In fact, no one could last more than a few minutes. When they threw in the towel, Jones measured heart rates, blood pressure and other physical parameters. Nothing seemed abnormal, although it was obvious that the demand was more than the body could handle. Jones speculated that the intensity and pace of the effort exceeded the body's ability to keep stride with necessary chemical changes which prompted a state of "shock." Ironically, he considered the intensity and pace *prerequisites* for "best" results from exercise. The body could, and would eventually, adapt to handle the demand.

Jones' early work focused on muscle size and strength. Impressed by the results produced with Viator in 1971, professional bodybuilders Sergio Oliva, Boyer Coe, Ray and Mike Mentzer and Dorian Yates jumped on the "high-intensity" bandwagon. In 1973 Jones hired Ellington Darden, a bodybuilder and recent graduate of Florida State University with a Doctorate in nutrition. Darden was intrigued by Jones' persona and novel ideas; it helped his progress. He began to write books that defined the Nautilus philosophy of exercise, providing structure to theory and application to a wider audience. By the mid-1970's focus had shifted to the athletic community where roots had already been established.

In 1972 Miami Dolphins' coach Don Shula took an interest in Jones' work and, on the back of the new system, coached his team to the only undefeated season in NFL history. Interest was further heightened by the results of "Project Total Conditioning" conducted at West Point Academy in 1975 with members of the U.S. Army's collegiate teams (notably football, wrestling and volleyball). Shula was still involved and witnessed the experiment that by now covered all five aspects of conditioning—strength, flexibility, cardiovascular, injury prevention and body composition.

Let it be clear: Progressive resistance exercise performed under ANY guidelines, in reasonable form, will increase strength and simultaneously improve the status of its by-products—body composition and injury protection. Flexibility can increase with the proper use of free-weights or machines but requires special attention to form—an attention generally absent in gyms. Cardiovascular ability is the single potential benefit that is *not* automatically produced with just ANY form of resistance training, which is why it is often treated as a separate entity. Proper Strength Training is the only system to include the cardiovascular component by reducing time between exercises, thereby satisfying the requirements of all five potential benefits.

In plain English, Proper Strength Training can do it all and do it better.

CHAPTER 3

Potential Benefits of Exercise

...Properly performed exercise is capable of producing far better results than most people even suspect . . . so since you are spending the time and making the investment, why not get the best results you can?

Arthur Jones

There are five potential benefits of exercise: an increase in strength, flexibility and cardiovascular condition; an improvement in body composition; and a decrease in the possibility of injury. The act of performing exercise, however, does not ensure any of the above: All five are *indirect* results. That is, exercise stimulates change and the body makes the change at its leisure. The only *direct* result of exercise is injury, which occurs the moment a muscle/joint system is exposed to a force that exceeds its structural integrity—and that change is instant.

Productive exercise, then, carries two burdens: It must stimulate change and, at the same time, keep the forces involved in check. The first is accomplished by challenging the body to surpass existing limits. The second deals with proper execution—exercise form.

In broad terms, exercise can be divided into two varieties: steady-state and non steady-state. The former relates to prolonged efforts traditionally associated with stimulating the cardiovascular system—cycling, running, swimming, etc. The proper application of steady-state exercise addresses two of the five benefits. Non steady-state exercise refers to brief, intense efforts typically linked to stimulating the muscular system—strength training. Its proper application can effectively satisfy all five, as follows . . .

Strength

Skeletal muscles require stimulation to increase and/or maintain size and strength. Progressive resistance exercise provides the means. The stimulation required *to maintain* existing levels involves the repetition of a physical task at regular intervals, while the stimulation required *to surpass* existing levels involves forcing a muscle to do something above and beyond the "norm"—which sends a different signal. If that signal repeats, the body adjusts its dials to the new level of stress and stringently guards a reserve for future or emergency use. The muscles involved (and the body to a lesser degree) become stronger and remain so as long as signals continue to arrive.

Each muscle has a "threshold of stimulation," a level of work intensity that triggers an adaptive signal. Intensity below this value has little to no effect on change; intensity at or above initiates the adaptive process—turns the switch "ON." To date, science has confirmed the threshold's existence and its variation from muscle to muscle within the same individual—but has struggled with its *exact* quantification. Thousands of studies on fiber-type have determined that muscles with a predominance of "fast-twitch" (strong, powerful) fibers require a lower number of repetitions to reach their threshold, whereas muscles with a predominance of "slow-twitch" (weaker, endurance) fibers require a higher repetition scheme to stimulate growth. Arthur Jones studied the phenomenon with rehabilitation tools he developed in 1986 and determined that a reduction of one's starting strength by approximately 20% due to exercise created an "ideal" stimulus regardless of fiber-type. He also believed that a muscle's threshold of stimulation represented a high percentage of its momentary ability; and that a greater recruitment of muscle fibers was directly related to effort (intensity)—the key to stimulating change.

Specific threshold values may never be determined, which may prove irrelevant. If you knew, for example, that your biceps required a 96% effort to create a stimulus for growth, how would you produce it during exercise?

There's no bell to go off. The only way you can be assured of reaching *any* threshold value is to perform work at 100% of your capacity, until the muscle cannot complete a full repetition—a state Jones called "momentary muscle failure."

In other words, **exercise for the purpose of gaining strength must be hard . . .**

. . . and **must be progressive**. The stimulus must continue to challenge the muscle to exceed its limits. Progress is defined by increasing the load to which a muscle is exposed or increasing the number of repetitions performed with the same load. True progress is achieved when either or both are increased and all other components of form (speed of movement, body position, range of motion, etc.) remain constant.

. . . and **must involve as great a range of motion as possible**.

"The best type of exercise is one that involves full range movement, movement that starts from a fully extended, pre-stretched position and continues to a fully contracted position. Anything less than a full-range movement will provide exercise for only part of a muscle, and will do little or nothing in the way of improving flexibility." [1]

An increase in muscle strength is generally accompanied by an increase in size—larger muscles are required to handle the greater demand. But while the prospect of larger muscles provides the fuel to exercise for males, it often turns females away. Without going into detail, everyone is capable of increasing strength to a degree they may have thought impossible and that alone will increase functional ability. But *not* everyone is capable of increasing muscle size to the same degree. The potential for size is genetic and *few* have the potential depicted in bodybuilding publications. Estimates for males are one in a million; females, one in ten million.

Over the years, I have met the majority of female exceptions.

"At this point in time," said Jones, *"nobody seriously claims to know exactly why a muscle responds to exercise by growing stronger. But we do know how to produce this result. Practical experience has clearly and repeatedly*

established the fact that proper exercise is capable of producing literally enormous increases in muscular strength. And practical experience has also established the fact that no amount of low-intensity exercise will produce the results that come from an actually small amount of high-intensity training. We can conjecture to our heart's content about exactly why this is so, but in the meantime we can also make good practical application of the fact that it is so." [2]

Cardiovascular

The strength of muscle contraction is the only thing that produces human movement. A contracting muscle requires oxygen; and repeated contractions, more. Oxygen is supplied by the circulatory system, directed by the nervous system and pumped by the heart—a heart that is not particularly smart. Other than volume and rate differences, it cannot distinguish between an arm and a leg. A signal is sent; the heart responds. If signals are brief, as in non steady-state exercise, the heart delivers what it must and quickly initiates a recovery phase to reassume its normal state. If signals are prolonged, as during steady-state exercise, the heart adjusts its rate and volume to equal the demand. According to research an effort of twelve minutes or more that sustains your heart rate within parameters (defined primarily by age) provides a stimulus to the heart to adapt or maintain. If the stimulus is of sufficient intensity and duration—and frequently applied—the effect is an increase in the efficiency and effectiveness of all related systems (heart, lung, circulatory, etc.).

Cardiovascular ability is an absolute requirement for life. For that, and because it is a common medical recommendation, traditional cardiovascular exercise (treadmills, bikes, elliptical trainers, etc.) is the most popular choice in gyms. It is simple, easily measured and efficient. An increase in cardiovascular fitness generally triggers an increase in the performance of sports and activities of daily living. An exceptional cardiovascular capacity may define the difference between "mediocre" and a world champion.

Many sports themselves provide the requirements of cardiovascular exercise. Frequent swimming, for example, can develop the condition required to swim—the same with soccer, field hockey and basketball. Nonetheless, many athletes in these sports also partake in supplemental cardiovascular training, whether by demand or by choice. When I coached men's soccer at Averett College in Virginia (1972-76), I ran seven to ten miles three times a week. Playing a full game was not a challenge.

Cardiovascular exercise, it seems, receives the attention it deserves from sports and fitness—but not in an efficient manner. In fitness settings, trainees pressed for time do it almost exclusively—a mistake. Treadmills, elliptical trainers and bikes do NOT strengthen the major muscle structures of the body: They exercise the heart alone. Trainees *not* pressed for time generally perceive it as something apart from muscle training. They don't associate the two—another natural mistake. A strength-training program, properly designed, can elicit a cardiovascular response that equals or surpasses that achieved through traditional means.

In a recent review of research that referenced 157 studies, a group from Britain and the United States investigated the effect of resistance training on the cardiovascular system. The "differences" drawn from previous studies between short-term and long-term effects of traditional aerobic training versus resistance training were inconclusive due to, for the most part, a failure to identify the intensity of exercise. The research itself, however, appeared *"to support the recommendation that resistance training (whether circuit style or traditional, and independent of other resistance training variables) performed to failure is sufficient to induce significant improvement in cardiovascular fitness."* Strength training continued to momentary muscle fatigue, the review concluded, *". . . can induce acute and chronic physiological effects which appear to be similar to aerobic endurance training, which in turn produces similar enhancements in cardiovascular fitness."* [3]

The key to stimulating the cardiovascular system through progressive resistance exercise, according to the review, was *"intense muscular contraction,"* which explains the extraordinary cardiovascular results produced by the intense strength training during "Project Total Conditioning" in 1975 (outlined in Chapter 14). The results of the experiment conducted by Jones and measured by Dr. Kenneth Cooper's elite team, stunned the field of exercise but failed to impress those who remained firm in their belief that Arthur was blowing smoke. Apparently he wasn't.

Flexibility

Exercise should and can increase flexibility—but it seldom does. Flexibility is increased *during* exercise under two conditions: ONE, that exercise is performed over a full range of motion; and TWO, that resistance is involved when a muscle reaches the limits of its extended (versus flexed) position.

Strength training and muscle size are often falsely associated with losses in flexibility—a perception quickly dismissed by comparing two groups of athletes. Gymnasts are muscular, yet flexible; runners are slighter and less muscular, but inflexible. Gymnastics demands a great range of motion about the joints, while the action of running is mid-range. John Grimek, a bodybuilder from the 1940's and described as "one of the bulkiest muscular men in history," could touch his elbows to the floor from a standing position with his legs locked at the knees, perform full splits, and assume positions far beyond the norm. *"You can lift weights,"* he said, *"and be called muscle-bound, and not lift weights and actually be muscle-bound."* Large muscles are unrelated to flexibility or its lack.

Exercise that involves stretching will increase flexibility; exercise that does not involve stretching will not increase (or maintain) flexibility. NO stretching can occur when exercise is performed through a mid or partial range of motion, or when no resistance is applied to the working muscle in a stretched position.

A stretch occurs when a muscle exceeds its existing range of motion within the confines of the joint system. Most conventional exercises do NOT provide a stretch when the muscle reaches an extended position—which makes exercise selection important. Many bodybuilders believe that a traditional barbell bench press, for example, stretches the muscles of the chest and front shoulder, and that a wider grip provides a greater stretch. Wrong. Bench-press movements are blocked by the chest and a wide grip further restricts the range of motion (by as much as twenty-one degrees). By comparison, a dip works the same muscles but allows a deeper stretch—a greater range of motion—and would be a better choice for flexibility, properly performed.

> **You can lift weights and be called muscle-bound, and not lift weights and actually be muscle-bound.**

As typically performed, however, dips are non-productive and often dangerous. Trainees use too much weight, lower themselves halfway down, bounce back using a fast speed and wonder why strength results are slow at best, why their shoulders hurt and why they lose flexibility. Form is as important as exercise selection. A muscle must approach a position that challenges the limits of its ability to stretch at a SLOW speed. A fast approach triggers a reflex contraction that prohibits a stretch—for safety.

Properly performed, some conventional exercises provide a stretch: dips, shoulder shrugs, dead lifts from a bench, triceps curls on an incline bench, full squats, heel raises on a step and wrist curls on a decline bench. But few provide resistance when a muscle reaches an extended position. Machines that provide a direct, variable and balanced resistance to muscles through a full range of motion are the exception. Properly performed, these tools better meet the requirements of an increase in flexibility during exercise . . . and in no small way.

A study conducted using two groups of college football players revealed the difference in flexibility gains between free-weight and machine training, as described:

During the course of an extensive research program conducted at the United States Military Academy, West Point, in April and May of 1975, two groups of varsity football players were compared on the basis of changes in flexibility produced by different styles of training.

Both groups of subjects were involved in spring football practice during the course of the experiment, and both groups were exposed to the normal stretching exercises that form part of a football practice . . . and both groups were involved in strength training programs, but here there was a difference.

One group was trained exclusively on Nautilus equipment . . . trained very briefly but very hard; a total of only seventeen brief workouts during a period of six weeks . . . workouts that averaged less than thirty minutes each.

Both groups were carefully tested before and after the period of training . . . and both groups improved their flexibility as a result of their training, but they did not improve equally.

In the first area of flexibility improvement, the Nautilus group improved ten times as much as the conventional group . . . not ten percent more, but ten times as much, literally a 1,000 percent increase.

In the second area of improvement, the Nautilus group improved eleven times as much as the conventional group, a 1,100 percent increase.

And in the third area, the Nautilus group improved more than twenty times as much as the conventional group, more than a 2,000 percent increase.

And, at the same time, while greatly improving their flexibility, the Nautilus trained subjects also increased in strength an average of nearly 60 percent, in only six weeks, as a result of only seventeen brief workouts . . . a total training time of approximately eight hours.

So it is obvious that properly conducted strength training will increase both strength and flexibility . . . and will do so rapidly.[4]

. . . so much for sprawling on the floor.

Body Composition

Fitness trainers generally focus on two components: muscle tissue and body fat. Their relationship (expressed as a muscle-mass/body-fat ratio) is dynamic and influenced by a simple formula—*Calories In: Calories Out.* Despite the claims of millions of products, input and output are the only valid tools we have to control body composition. Input is managed by diet; output, by metabolism and exercise.

A single pound of body fat contains 3,500 calories. A dietary reduction of 500 calories per day results in the loss of one pound of fat per week—*if other factors remain the same.* Nutrition expert, Ellington Darden, Ph.D. dedicated several of the early Nautilus books to diet/exercise programs aimed at reducing body fat. His dietary recommendations revolved around a daily caloric intake of 1,200-1,400 for women and 1,500-1,600 for men; a balanced intake of fat, protein and carbohydrates at every caloric level; and an altered total intake every two weeks to prevent stagnation.

The guidelines of his books, *32 Days to a 32-Inch Waist* and *The Six-Week Fat-to-Muscle Makeover* defined a fat-loss program we used in a facility in Wellington, Florida with great success.

Output offers two choices: steady-state and non steady-state exercise. With the average trainee and similar intensities, both burn calories at a rate of approximately 200 per half hour. There the similarity ends. The expenditure of calories during steady-state (aerobic) exercise results in "indiscriminate weight loss"—bodyweight lost from muscle, organ tissue *and* fat tissue—which means ten pounds lost while jogging comes from all sources. You don't want to lose muscle or organ tissue, just fat—which is why Dr. Darden did not recommend or allow *any* cardiovascular exercise during his programs.

Progressive resistance exercise, on the other hand, sends a signal to maintain or increase muscle integrity. The body responds by doing what it can to *prevent* muscle loss and increase metabolic demand. Every pound of muscle gained through strength training requires an additional expenditure of 50-100 calories per day to maintain itself. Since an average woman can add two to three pounds of muscle to her body in six weeks (an average man, three to four pounds in a month), the extra expenditure can result in 100-300 calories per day for females (and 150-400 for males). Both types of exercise (steady-state and non steady-state) burn calories before, during and after exercise; but only strength training creates prolonged metabolic activity. Weeks after, new muscle still demands breakfast.

Of the two (diet and exercise), a reduction in calories produces a quicker response. Burning calories by output alone can be a slow and arduous process—especially if the choice is steady-state exercise. Three half-hour cardiovascular workouts per week—at 200 calories per session—results in a loss of one pound of body fat every 17½ sessions, about six weeks.

Proper strength training is quicker. In *The Nautilus Diet Book* (1987), Darden supervised approximately 100 subjects (male, female, young and old) and produced the following results during a ten-week program: an **average fat loss** of 18.75 pounds (women) and 30.0 pounds (men); and an average muscle gain of 2.5 pounds (women) and 4.0 pounds (men). The book featured complete measurements and before/after photos of *every* person in the study. And again, no aerobic exercise was performed.

An aside: *On the extreme end of body-composition modification was 1971 Mr. America, Casey Viator who demonstrated the role of genetics in the process. Viator was blessed with an outstanding potential for muscle mass. In January of 1973 he was involved in an industrial accident in which he nearly lost the little finger of his right hand, almost died from an allergic reaction to a tetanus shot, lost thirty-three pounds of bodyweight and sat around depressed. Jones, who had trained Viator for the 1971 competition, flew a set of Nautilus machines to Fort Collins, Colorado and arranged a strength-training "experiment" directed by Dr. Elliot Plese, Ph.D. of the exercise physiology department. Casey performed one set each of twelve exercises to failure, every other day for twenty-eight days and produced the following results: a bodyweight gain of 45.28 pounds (from 166.87 to 212.15); a body-fat loss of 17.93 pounds; a body-fat percentage drop from 13.8 to 2.47; and a net muscle gain of 63.21 pounds in fourteen workouts. Although it was obvious that Viator was "rebuilding previously existing levels of muscular size," the experiment represented an outstanding example of what can be accomplished with "freakish" genes and proper strength training.*

Thirty years of observation has led me to believe that trainees seeking to reduce their waistlines make poor choices—cardiovascular choices—because it's simple and often indentifies caloric expenditure. At the same time, they ignore strength training because it makes them "weigh more." Let it be clear: It is easily possible to lose strength while gaining weight or gain strength while losing weight. Don't judge results by the scale; judge by how clothes fit. Focus on body fat, not body weight. And have your body-composition measured by a professional at regular intervals to check progress.

Strength training is the most effective and efficient way to modify your body's external aesthetics and internal composition.

Every pound of muscle gained through strength training requires an additional expenditure of 50-100 calories per day to maintain itself.

Protection from Injury

Common sense prevailed with Arthur Jones, *". . . exercise can greatly reduce the chances of injury, but exercise is also capable of causing injury. The best type of exercise is the type that is most likely to prevent injury, and least likely to cause injury."*

The difference between cause and prevention lies in execution—how exercise is performed. Injury is a tug-of-war between two factors: structural integrity and external force. If a muscle/joint structure of 100-units strong is exposed to a force of 101 units, something breaks. Injury prevention offers two choices: increase the integrity of the structure or decrease the force to which it is exposed. The first is the purpose of progressive resistance training—increase the strength of the muscles surrounding the joint to enhance function and decrease the chance of injury. The second is misunderstood.

Resistance

Most trainees believe that the use of heavy weights and high intensity promotes injury. Their solution—to reduce both resistance and effort—may be a safe option, but it is far from productive and not the BEST way to prevent injury. The "heaviness" of a weight is relative. If you walk "untrained" into a gym to compete with your buddies on a bench press or select a resistance that compromises form, you're asking for trouble. On the contrary, if you increase the weight you lift for ten repetitions from 250 to 255 pounds, have gradually progressed to that point and do not change form, you will NOT injure yourself regardless of how close the weight is to your strength potential.

Form

Jones believed that two ingredients produced best results from exercise: good form and high intensity. Most people understand the first—but don't practice what they preach. Good form begins with a slow speed of movement, as noted:

Jerky movements are directly responsible for a very high percentage of the injuries caused by exercise, and jerky movements are of little or no value for the purpose of developing strength. Exercises performed for the purpose of increasing strength should always be smooth. Sudden movements and rapid accelerations should be avoided.[5]

Fast, jerky movements elevate the force to which a muscle is exposed. A 100-pound barbell moved in an explosive manner can expose working muscles to a force in excess of 300 pounds. In contrast, slow, controlled movements keep the forces involved very near the actual value of the weight being lifted and challenge muscles to "lift" rather than "throw" weight. It only takes a force of 101 pounds to move a 100-pound resistance.

Intensity

High levels of intensity are counterintuitive. When trainees reach the end of a tough set, they generally back off because they have satisfied a pre-set quota or believe that it is somehow dangerous. It may "feel" as if your arms are about to fall off or thighs explode as you reach momentary muscle failure, but it doesn't tell the entire story:

. . . a high level of force (resistance) is not required for high intensity. In fact, if exercises are performed properly, then the maximum intensity repetitions will actually involve less force. It is easily possible and very desirable to have high intensity and low force at the same time. A failure to understand this simple point has led to a ridiculous situation that is very commonly encountered in exercise programs.

Many, perhaps most, trainees avoid the final two or three repetitions in a set under the totally mistaken belief that they are avoiding the most dangerous repetitions. In fact, the final repetitions are actually the safest, because the output is lower, the production of force is lower. During the final repetition

---

A 100-pound barbell moved in an explosive manner can expose working muscles to a force in excess of 300 pounds.

---

the trainee is imposing less pulling force on his muscular attachments than he was during the first few repetitions. In practice, thousands of trainees avoid the most productive repetitions under the false impression that they are thus avoiding the dangerous repetitions. But they have already performed the most dangerous repetitions, the first few repetitions, and are actually skipping the safest repetitions. As a direct consequence, most trainees produce results that are far below optimum results, because a very high percentage of the strength increases produced by exercise is a direct result of high intensity, which is involved only in the final two or three repetitions.

Several years of exercise that is stopped three repetitions short of a point of momentary failure will not produce results equal to those that can be produced in a matter of a few weeks by an otherwise exactly similar training program that is carried to the point of momentary failure.

The first two or three repetitions are merely preparation and do little or nothing in the way of increasing strength. These repetitions are of little value because the intensity is low. The final repetitions are productive because the intensity is high.

Since the facts in this case, simple and undeniable though they are, run contrary to the widespread belief, it will be a long time before this point is understood and accepted by a high percentage of trainees or coaches. In the meantime, most strength programs will consist primarily of wasted effort. Millions of man-hours of training and billions of foot-pounds of effort will be devoted to programs that produce little if anything of value.[6]

Safety during exercise depends on the momentary capability of the muscle to produce force. When a muscle is fresh at the start of a set, it is capable of producing high levels of force but should NOT—and a slow, controlled speed of movement will ensure that it CANNOT. At the end of a set, an exhausted muscle is incapable of producing a force high enough to break anything. High levels of intensity during exercise create a safer work environment for the muscle, produce superior strength results and better protect the body from injury.

Food for Thought

The potential benefits of exercise are fleeting—a common complaint among trainees and a convenient excuse for non-trainees. *"In general,"* says Arthur Jones, *"the longer you maintain a high level of strength, the more you will retain after you quit the exercise that increased your strength in the first place."* If strength is acquired or maintained briefly—and exercise terminated—trainees might expect a rapid loss of eighty to one-hundred percent of their gains. A strength increase acquired or maintained for two years, on the other hand, might result in a loss of only fifty to sixty percent upon cessation.

This phenomenon of loss extends to all five potential benefits of exercise to some degree or another—but there is good news: When you return to exercise, previous peak levels of conditioning are more readily attained. The body has memory that allows it to reach previous levels of condition faster than it initially did.

The traditional approach to exercise focuses on single benefits: Strength training for strength, aerobic training for cardiovascular condition and stretching for flexibility. It also regards body-composition and injury-prevention as tagalongs—something that happens as a result of the rest. Few training regimens address multiple benefits and few trainees regard a single system as "complete."

Arthur Jones believed otherwise. He thought all five benefits could be acquired by one style of exercise—Proper Strength Training—a system that had local *and* global ramifications, as described:

"Properly performed exercise will improve the condition, the overall system of any athlete. The conditioning results of exercise are produced regardless of what part of the human structure is being exercised. Working the arms has exactly the same effect on the heart and lungs as exercise involving the legs if the total amount of work and the pace are the same. The heart and lungs do not know which muscles are working. Foot-pounds of work performed and the pace of training are all that matter for conditioning purposes.

But strength increases are specific to a high degree. Heavy exercise performed for the right arm will do very little for the left arm and almost nothing for the legs. While it is true that some degree of lateral effect does occur, it is very limited in its results. Lateral effect is growth produced in, for example, an unworked left arm by exercise performed by the right arm.

It is also true that an even greater degree of indirect effect is also produced by exercise. But again, it is limited in its results. Indirect effect is growth produced in one muscular structure as a result of exercise performed by other muscles.

However, if we accept the limited results of lateral effect and indirect effect, then the strength increases resulting from exercise are almost entirely specific in nature. Work must be performed by the muscle the athlete is attempting to strengthen.

. . . the conditioning results of exercise are general and the strength increasing results are specific.

. . . Steady-state training (aerobic exercise) will never produce much in the way of meaningful strength increases, and non steady-state training (strength exercise, as commonly performed) will do little or nothing for cardiovascular ability. However, a particular muscle can be worked to a point of momentary muscular failure in a very brief period of time, in a non steady-state fashion, and then another muscle can be worked immediately.

If the program is outlined properly, every major muscle group in the body can be worked in a non steady-state fashion (for strength), while training the system as a whole in a steady-state (aerobic) fashion.

This is not merely a theory. It works. It works far better than any other style of training that we have ever tried, and we have tried everything we ever heard of that seemed to offer even the possibility of worthwhile results, and quite a number of things that were obviously of no possible value." [7]

REFERENCES

[1] Jones, A., "What to Expect from Exercise," Peterson, J.A., Ph.D. (editor), *Total Fitness the Nautilus Way*, Leisure Press, 3: 42, 1978.

[2] Jones, A., "What to Expect from Exercise," Peterson, J.A., Ph.D. (editor), *Total Fitness the Nautilus Way*, Leisure Press, 3: 46, 1978.

[3] Steele, J., Fisher, J., McGuff, D., Bruce-Low, S., Smith, D., "Resistance Training to Momentary Muscular Failure Improves Cardiovascular Fitness in Humans: A Review of Acute Physiological Responses and Chronic Physiological Adaptations," *Journal of Exercise Physiology online*, 15-3 June, 2012.

[4] Jones, A., "Flexibility as a Result of Exercise," Peterson, J.A., Ph.D. (editor), *Total Fitness the Nautilus Way*, Leisure Press, 18: 188-190, 1978.

[5] Jones, A., "What to Expect from Exercise," Peterson, J.A., Ph.D. (editor), *Total Fitness the Nautilus Way*, Leisure Press, 3: 42, 1978.

[6] Jones, A., "Progressive Exercise," Peterson, J.A., Ph.D. (editor), *Total Fitness the Nautilus Way*, Leisure Press, 4: 48-50, 1978.

[7] Jones, A., "What to Expect from Exercise," Peterson, J.A., Ph.D. (editor), *Total Fitness the Nautilus Way*, Leisure Press, 3: 35-44, 1978.

....

CHAPTER 4

Strength Training Principles

"Everything of value related to exercise can be stated in less than a thousand words, can, in fact, be fairly well covered in a few words, as follows: Train hard, train briefly, train infrequently."

Arthur Jones

On The Bus

The establishment of strength training principles is far from "a science." Fuzzy research, questionable conclusions, pseudo-scientific publications and the opinions of a myriad of certification groups have resulted in a pile of confusion dumped on a public scratching their heads about "how to get the job done." How many sets? How many repetitions? How often? How fast? How slow?

Where do you turn for *valid* information?

Dave Smith and Stewart Bruce-Low of the Department of Sport and Exercise Sciences at the University of Liverpool in England made a start. They reviewed exercise-physiology textbooks, strength-and-conditioning journals and popular certification guidelines[1] to extract the following consensus on how to produce optimum results from strength training—ideas in current use:

- Perform multiple sets of each exercise.
- Apply low-repetition sets to increase strength and high-repetition sets to increase muscular endurance.

- Perform explosive repetitions to develop optimum power.
- Experienced trainees should perform more exercise, up to four to five days per week, twice a day for a total of up to twenty-one hours per week.

The Brits disagreed with what they found—and were not alone. Two independent review articles[2] that followed supported opposite views and confirmed the longstanding feud between high-volume and high-intensity exercise.

High-volume training has been around as long as its critics. In December, 2004, Smith and Bruce-Low published an article in the *Journal of the American Society of Exercise Physiologists* titled: "Strength Training Methods and the Work of Arthur Jones." It recognized the contributions of a major critic.

Off the Bus

The pair began by examining three of Jones' books (*Nautilus Training Principles, Bulletin No. 1.,* 1970; *Bulletin No 2.,* 1971; and *The Lumbar Spine,* 1988) and more than 100 of his published articles. His recommendations were unique:

- Perform one set of each exercise to muscular failure.
- Work each muscle group no more than twice a week.
- Move slowly and smoothly during each repetition.
- Perform eight to twelve repetitions for optimal increases in muscle strength *and* endurance.

The concepts were backed by practical experience, logical thinking, the laws of physics and a brilliant mind—but were, nonetheless, ridiculed and tossed aside. They threatened the status quo and were *never* afforded a scientific critique—until recently.

Number of Sets

Beginning in 2004 Smith and Bruce-Low reviewed forty-one studies that compared single versus multiple sets, examining ambiguity in variables, experimenter bias, statistics and conclusions, as well as planning and accurate reporting. They found that many of the references cited in books and articles were NOT research studies or scientific evidence, but opinion, and determined, "*. . . that the great majority of well controlled, peer-reviewed studies support Jones' contention that one set to failure is all that is necessary to stimulate optimal increases in muscular size and strength.*"

The findings reflect the results of research conducted at the University of Florida in the mid 1990's. In the midst of "doing their three-set thing," the research staff at the Center for Exercise Science eventually gave in to Jones' insistence that *"one set is enough."* They reviewed every study that compared one set to multiple sets from 1962 and, regardless of outcome, found no result "statistically significant." They then conducted their own study with the recently-developed MedX Medical Knee machine by testing (and exercising) the front-thigh and rear-thigh strength of two large groups of untrained subjects. They found that one set of exercise to failure produced the *same* strength increase as three sets to failure with both muscle groups. The results were measured on a machine that took twenty years to perfect at a cost of $120 million. There was no question about accuracy.

Exercise Frequency

Smith and Bruce-Low examined ten studies related to exercise frequency and found that training each muscle twice a week produces optimal results.

> The great majority of well controlled, peer-reviewed studies support Jones' contention that one set to failure is all that is necessary to stimulate optimal increases in muscular size and strength.

Speed of Movement

They reviewed twenty studies that dealt with speed of movement and, contrary to the consensus that "explosive" training is superior for strength and power, found two alternatives: that slow training was *superior* to explosive training (to develop strength and power) or, that there was *no significant difference* between slow and fast speeds. More important, four other studies they cited reported the serious risk of injury from explosive training. The researchers concluded, *"It appears that Jones' recommendation that slow, controlled weight training is all that is necessary to enhance both muscular strength and power is correct."*

Number of Repetitions

Eight studies related to repetition range revealed that low-to-moderate schemes produced both optimal results and proportionate increases in strength *and* muscular endurance. Low-repetition ranges did NOT produce better strength gains but demonstrated a greater inherent danger to joint and connective tissue. High-repetition ranges were of NO value to the production of muscle endurance. A range of eight to twelve (8-12) was deemed *"effective and prudent."*

The concepts of Arthur Jones were *scientifically* validated by the work of Smith and Bruce-Low—but it failed to tip the scales: The majority of trainers and trainees are still "on the bus," with few willing to get off—and more buses added every day.

Let's move on . . .

High-repetition ranges were of NO value to the production of muscle endurance.

The force of muscle contraction creates movement. And whether that movement manifests itself in reaching the dining hall at the nursing home or in a world-class performance, strength makes it happen and provides a hidden benefit: Strength increases the integrity of the system that delivers the product. And that allows movement to proceed more efficiently, quickly (if needed), with less effort and in a safer environment—a good "deal."

Unfortunately, the "deal" has been undermined by faulty training technique, lack of understanding and, of late, an influx of exercise choices that water-down and confuse the issue.

Throughout the 1970's and 1980's Arthur Jones trained some of the strongest individuals on the planet—athletes, bodybuilders and world-class competitors—and reduced the principles of Proper Strength Training to a handful of ideas related to intensity, form and progression.

Intensity

◄ The intensity of effort must be high to stimulate change.

Jones believed that most trainees performed too much exercise. When he questioned first-timers to the Nautilus facility about training habits, they generally rattled off a list as long as their arm. He responded by housing them for days in a remote motel along the beach, far from the possibility of exercise. When he brought them in to train, a second belief was confirmed: Few worked hard. The missing link was intensity, and that belief was not a first:

More than a century ago, by a study of the bones of men who spent their lives at manual labor, it was determined that the intensity of work is a factor of great importance; even the chemical composition of the bones is changed by hard work. How much you work—the actual "amount" of work—is a factor of only secondary importance, and then usually in a negative sense. In effect, "hard work" is a desirable factor—and a large "amount of work" is an undesirable factor.[3]

A high level of intensity is a prerequisite to stimulate muscle growth, but it can only be measured under two circumstances: during zero effort and during a 100-percent effort. Zero effort is of no value to exercise; 100% paves the way to growth stimulation, efficiency and safety.

Intensity is effort—a percentage of momentary ability. Maximum intensity occurs when a muscle is producing as much pulling force as it momentarily can. When that occurs, the muscle recruits more of its fibers *and* its largest fibers to the effort. Their involvement increases the odds of gaining strength.

At the practical level maximum intensity manifests itself in two ways: ONE, reaching "momentary muscle failure" during exercise—the inability to move against resistance despite a full effort; and TWO, resting less between efforts. The process is neither easy nor pretty. Funny faces, color changes and increased post-effort recovery attest to a degree of difficulty that few are willing to explore.

◣ Intensity dictates the duration and frequency of workouts.

If you work HARD, you won't last long—a physical fact. Workouts must be brief—and will be—if the effort required to stimulate change is employed. And that defines the mission of exercise: Maximum muscle stimulation with minimal effect on the system's recovery ability. With harder work, the system requires more time to recover and, logically, less stimulation frequency.

◣ High-intensity exercise greatly decreases the possibility of injury.

When a muscle reaches failure, its strength has been diminished to the point that it is no longer capable of producing a force high enough to exceed structural limits, which makes the final repetitions of a set the *least* likely to cause injury.

Form

"Ninety-five percent of the people in this country who perform progressive resistance exercise," the Nautilus inventor commented, *"do not know how*

> Workouts must be brief - and will be - if the effort required to stimulate change is employed.

to lift or lower one repetition of any exercise." From the side of his mouth, he'd add, *"More like 99.9."* The estimate may be conservative. Everyone talks "good form," but few do it or know how to.

◖ Good form requires proper exercise position.

Set seats at proper heights on machines and fasten seat belts (if provided) to better target the muscle(s) trained. Align your joint system with the rotational axis of the machine (where possible). Assume a secure exercise posture before you begin and assure that your station is clear of hazards.

◖ Good form begins with a SLOW speed of movement that keeps tension on the muscle throughout the exercise.

A slow speed of movement makes exercise HARDER: Anything that makes exercise harder makes it more productive. How slow?—a speed that allows you to "feel" the weight and that makes the muscle "work" during *every* part of the movement. Most trainees are surprised by how slow that is.

To add, a slow speed during exercise decreases the chance of injury.

Progression

◖ Try to increase repetitions or resistance during each workout, but keep your repetition range at eight to twelve.

Good results from strength training require an attempt to make progress during every workout. A muscle will not grow without stimulation, and stimulation can only occur when a muscle is challenged to exceed its current limits.

In the early 1970's a repetition scheme of eight to twelve was thought to produce best results from strength training. That hasn't changed. If you cannot perform eight repetitions in good form, the weight is too heavy. If you can perform twelve or more repetitions in good form, the weight should be increased by approximately 5% during the next workout.

- **Don't finish a set of exercise because you have reached twelve repetitions.**

Twelve is not a magic number. Continue until movement is no longer possible.

- **Never increase resistance at the expense of form.**

The body loves to play games. When you increase the weight of an exercise, the muscles sense the difference and respond predictably: "Let's move a little faster to reduce the burden." Within months, form that was once good and "established" deteriorates into something unrecognizable. Bad habits, often subconscious, nullify good intentions, which is why all trainees should have their form reviewed from time to time.

Apparently not all bad habits are subconscious.

A nice kid with a broad back entered my gym in Caracas in 1983. The self-proclaimed bodybuilder had heard about "Naw-tee-loose" (emphasis on the "tee"), had seen pictures in the magazines and was eager to start. He was sore after the first session but couldn't wait for the next. Things changed. Alejandro was so intent on using heavy weights that he began to "play the game." Unlike the majority of members who were "stuck" at eleven, he consistently performed twelve—and every time he did I increased the weight. One day I set him up on a machine and left to attend another client. When I returned (thirty seconds later), I asked, "How many?" He replied, "Twelve." I suspected that he didn't have time to do twelve good ones so I set him on the next machine, appeared to leave but lingered, and witnessed three repetitions.

"How many?"

"Twelve."

I jumped. He claimed a headache. So did I. The nice kid with the broad back did not return.

⬛ "Standardize" as many variables as possible.

True progress occurs when repetitions or weight are increased and as many variables as possible remain "standardized." The number of repetitions performed today may increase because the sequence is different. Variety is important, but it is equally important to retain a basic or favorite sequence that you perform every two weeks or every month so that valid comparisons can be made. Short of having access to exceptional testing tools, the only way to determine progress is to compare one performance with a previous performance **under the same conditions**. Ten repetitions today, **under the same conditions** of speed, sequence, time of day, resistance, etc. trumps nine repetitions performed two weeks prior.

⬛ Muscle Strength = Muscle Endurance.

Many trainees test their progress by checking how much they can lift one time, believing that the determination of peak strength from a performance of ten repetitions is more a test of muscle endurance. Without elaboration at this point, muscle strength and local muscular endurance are one and the same. An increase in one creates an equal increase in the other (as further discussed in Chapter 7). As a result of the misunderstanding, the standard test for muscle strength remains the performance of one repetition with as much resistance as possible (1RM—one repetition maximum)—a dangerous and inaccurate method. The demonstration of strength has nothing to do with the process of gaining strength. Unless you are a competitive weightlifter, strength can be safely and effectively determined by comparing two performances of an equal number of repetitions (ranging from eight to twelve). An accurate training record will help establish daily, weekly and long-term goals.

⬛ As strength continues to increase, perform less exercise.

Growth is rarely linear, as observed: *"The human muscular structure is capable of growing at an almost alarming rate, as has been clearly demonstrated in thousands of cases with beginning trainees. It was recently noted in the scientific community that growth occurs in very sudden spurts. A child may increase their height by as much as an inch overnight, literally in a few hours. I noticed the same thing in regard to gains in muscular size over 30 years ago: I have had my arms increase in size by a full inch from the time I went to bed at night until I got up the next morning, and while my increases in size have not always been that great, they have always been sudden, a matter of a few hours at most, and perhaps a matter of a few minutes. I was never able to determine just how much time was actually required for such spurts."* [4]

As we reach our strength potential, growth is often slow. In most cases this indicates lack of muscle stimulation or lack of systemic recovery. If the body's reserves are being constantly depleted by exercise, no growth can occur. The general workout frequency recommended for untrained subjects is three times per week. Following four to six months of training, the frequency MUST be reduced. The energy expenditure of workouts at that point creates a greater demand on the ability to recover. Less frequent training allows the body the time it needs to gather for future efforts.

Below (Figure 1) is a theoretical chart that demonstrates the progression from initial workout to strength potential. Note a *decrease* in the amount of exercise performed at each stage.

Figure 1: **REACHING STRENGTH POTENTIAL**

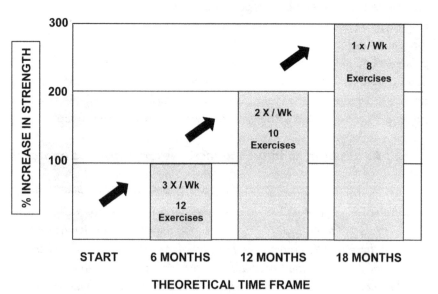

When Jones encountered plateaus, he ALWAYS reduced the amount of training, which allowed the system to better recover. In the end he believed his personal results would have improved had he reduced workouts to one brief session per week. Research agrees: Train each muscle twice a week, AT MOST, for best results.

Other Considerations

A few additional ideas to produce optimum results from strength training follow:

⚑ Work all the major structures of the body together.

Like comparing a "hard" punch to a "light" one, the system is better shocked to grow when all major muscles are worked together (in the same workout). The popular "split" routine (whereby trainees divide their body into parts) is the equivalent of sleeping for your thighs or eating for your calves.

Jones summed it up, *"For best results from exercise, all of the major muscle structures should be worked—ALL OF THEM, you certainly can build large arms without working your legs—but you will build them much larger, and much quicker, if you exercise your legs."* [5]

⚑ Select exercises that provide the greatest range of motion for the major muscle groups of the body (or the major muscles involved in your activity of interest).

In general, the larger the mass of muscle involved in an exercise, the greater the value of the exercise. If there is a choice, select exercises that move the targeted muscle through the greatest range of motion against resistance.

I had the good fortune to train Jack Nicklaus several times shortly after he had his hip replaced. I didn't want to go down in history as the man who screwed up the hip of the greatest golfer to ever play the game, so I sought the advice of a physical therapist. Besides caution with the hip the program focused on major muscle groups—thighs, hamstrings, glutes, calves, chest, shoulders, back and upper arms—and used the finest equipment, MedX®

machines. We sparingly trained the oblique muscles and those of the lumbar spine using MedX Medical tools as per protocol and performed occasional abdominal exercise on a machine. The focus was large, not small muscles.

One day as he warmed up, I asked Jack about the source of power in the golf swing. *"From the ground up,"* he replied—at a time when the majority of trainees (many, good golfers) and exercise programs in the media (television, magazines and books) focused on small muscles and made claims of reaching performance potential. Good luck.

> **◢ Perform one set of approximately twelve exercises: four to six for the lower-body (legs, hips); six to eight for the upper (torso, arms).**

Why twelve? When Jones first opened his commercial doors, the invitation to train was exactly that—"open." At the time he had only four "Nautilus Time Machines" available. The remaining stations featured Universal® machines or free-weights. Jones believed that one or two exercises per muscle group (twelve total sets for the body), properly performed, was enough to stimulate growth—and about all you could stand. He was right. The first person to finish the brief circuit—four years later—was the European cross-country ski champion. All others, including world-class athletes and bodybuilders, ended up on the floor despite, in some cases, a second and third attempt.

When I first opened shop in Caracas in 1980, I felt the same burden to prove the superiority of the system. Approximately thirty bodybuilders entered the first year and scoffed at my "hard-to-believe" introduction. When I challenged them to "give it a go," it was only a matter of time before they succumbed to the intensity and quick pace. ONE trainee made it to the fifth exercise; the others were on the floor or in the bathroom—in various states of disarray. It was not a fair fight.

From the beginning Jones sought to discover the minimum amount of exercise that produced the maximum result. Anything more was wasted effort at best and overtraining at worst. Without "official" research, he deemed one set of twelve exercises as a wise place to start.

☚ Work large muscles first and small muscles last, in sequence: Hips, legs, torso, arms, abdomen and others.

My gym in Venezuela was stark by design—the site had no barbells or dumbbells. One young man who was excited about the *new* training was discouraged by the fact that, when he reached the arm machines (near the end of the workout), he was so exhausted that he could not get much out of them. One day I rewarded his perseverance: *"Let's start with arms today and workout in reverse."* He couldn't contain his excitement. We started with a Nautilus Multi-Biceps machine and loaded it up—the kid was fresh. He tugged his gloves and dug in. Biceps, triceps, shoulders, back and chest—the kid was in heaven. When we reached the leg machines, I didn't expect or get much. Where he normally did ten repetitions, he got six. Twelve became eight; and nine, five. He had exhausted his systemic energy and could *not* perform the large-muscle exercises. Not his fault—the fault of poor program design. It's never a bad idea to "change things up," but it's important to exercise large muscles when you are "fresh." It hits the system harder.

☚ Perform brief workouts (twenty to thirty minutes with machines; thirty to forty-five with free weights).

If your workout is hard, it must be brief; if it is long, it can't be hard.

In the early years of Nautilus, three high-intensity workouts per week of approximately thirty minutes were recommended to everyone including professional bodybuilders. In some cases the reduction of weekly workout time from twenty-plus hours to ninety minutes was a shock, despite the fact that most couldn't make it. Jones eventually modified his stance to twice a week, a thirty-minute total. Results improved in general but the brief, infrequent training concepts were not embraced.

Today's trainees are more likely to accept a recommendation to perform four sets instead of three than a suggestion that points in the direction of *less* exercise. They can't connect *less* to more.

If your workout is hard, it must be brief; if it is long, it can't be hard.

🖦 **Allow a minimum of forty-eight hours (two days) and no more than ninety-six hours (four days) rest between workouts.**

The body is capable of performing any amount of exercise but not capable of recovering from any amount. The muscles *and* system require time to recover and adapt. Muscle recovery can be rapid, but systemic recovery (apart from how you "feel") is generally not—and the system feeds the muscles. When in doubt about frequency, err on the side of less.

🖦 **Move as quickly as you can from one exercise to the next as your condition improves.**

A rapid pace between exercises increases the intensity and cardiovascular component of a workout. If you opt to perform aerobic exercise apart from strength training, perform strength training first while you are fresh. It has more potential benefits than cardiovascular exercise. The *only* exception may be a trainee whose sport or medical condition prioritizes aerobic activity.

Summary

Below is a summary of strength training principles as they stood in the Nautilus heyday of the 1970's . . .

> - Perform one set of 12 exercises: 4-6 for the lower-body and 6-8 exercises for the upper-body.
> - Select a resistance that will allow 8-12 repetitions.
> - Continue each exercise to a point of momentary muscular failure.
> - When 12 or more repetitions are performed in perfect form, increase the resistance 5 percent during the next session.
> - Exercise larger muscle groups first and proceed to smaller.
> - Raise the weight to a two count; lower the weight to a four count. When in doubt about speed of movement, go slower.
> - Attempt to increase repetitions or resistance at every workout; but never sacrifice form in an attempt to get "one more rep."
> - Train no more than three times per week. Allow at least 48 hours, but no more than 96 hours, between workouts.
> - Keep accurate records: Date, resistance, repetitions and total workout time.
> - The entire workout should take 20-30 minutes.

. . . and as they stand today. The only alteration complies with what recent research demonstrates and with the final thoughts of Jones: Train no more than twice per week. With that, the principles of Proper Strength Training are defined and best framed by Arthur's pet phrase, *"We now know . . ."*

REFERENCES

[1] McArdle, W.D., Katch, F.I., Katch, V.L., *Exercise Physiology*, 2001; Wilmore, J.H., Costill, D.L., *Physiology of Sport and Exercise*, 1999; Bomba, T., *Serious Strength Training: Periodization for Building Muscle Power and Mass*, 1998; National Strength and Conditioning Association, *NSCA Position Statement 2003*; American College of Sports Medicine (ACSM), *Position Stand: Progressive Models in Resistance Training*, 2002.

[2] Carpinelli, R.N., Otto, R.M., Winett, R.A., "A Critical Analysis of the ACSM Position Stand on Resistance Training: Insufficient Evidence to Support Recommended Training Protocols," *Journal of Exercise Physiology online* 2004; 7 (3): 1-60; Winett, R.A., "Meta-Analyses Do Not Support Performance of Multiple Sets of High Volume Resistance Training," *Journal of Exercise Physiology online* 2004; 7 (5): 10-20.

[3] Jones, A., *Nautilus Training Principles Bulletin No. 2*, 26: 71, 1971.

[4] Jones, A., "My First Half Century in the Iron Game," *Ironman*: 7, 1973.

[5] Jones, A., *Nautilus Training Principles Bulletin No. 2*, 30: 85, 1971.

....

CHAPTER 5

Duration and Frequency

How much exercise is enough? The minimum that will produce the desired result should be used. Any exercise in excess of the minimum amount required will be wasted effort at best and counter-productive at the worst.

Arthur Jones

T he man who invented Nautilus machines spent a lifetime solving problems, connecting dots, establishing relationships between factors . . . and was good at it.

In the realm of exercise, he ONE, determined the strength potential of muscles at every angle of movement through a full range of motion by linking his knowledge of physics—leverage, angles of pull and moment arms—to his field work. The result was an "ideal" strength curve for an isolated muscle. When several muscles or joints were involved, he factored in the contribution of each (how much, when it appeared and how long it lasted) to determine an "ideal" strength curve for the movement. From that he created a "cam" that automatically delivered an ideal and variable resistance to the muscle or movement throughout its range of motion.

TWO, Jones established a relationship between strength and muscular endurance. He was able to determine his strength (how much he could lift one time) from the performance of ten repetitions. The ratio was unique and personal, but led to two important discoveries: that muscle strength could be determined without the use of a dangerous test; and, that muscle strength and muscle endurance were one and the same—a concept that remains foreign to most.

THREE, Jones established a relationship between lifting and lowering strength, attributing the difference to *internal muscle friction*, a phenomenon he eventually demonstrated and measured. It launched the acceptance of "negative work" as a viable means to stimulate growth.

Some of the relationships he exposed were "direct," others were "inverse" and a few were unkind. *"I don't believe,"* he said after training bodybuilders for years, *"that there is an inverse relationship between the size of a man's brain and the size of his biceps, but I'm beginning to suspect it."*

One "inverse" relationship was born of logic and practical experience: intensity versus duration. *"It must be clearly understood,"* he said, *"that high-intensity training and a large amount of training are mutually exclusive factors."* If you have one, you cannot have the other . . .

. . . and that made the choice clear: you either exercise brief and hard, or long and easy. Most advanced trainees prefer the latter—which has led to a consensus that you must "live" in the gym to get results. Not so. *"Twenty years ago,"* said Jones, *"I finally learned that an actual proper workout with barbells had to be brief in the extreme—so brief that I was always tempted to increase the number of exercises or sets, since the workout never appeared to contain 'enough;' but when I did increase anything in the workouts, the production of results was always reduced, ALWAYS."* [1]

The concept applies to all physical efforts. You can run 100 meters full-out but cannot if you extend the distance. At 400 meters or four miles you must pace yourself: The longer the run, the slower the pace.

Strength training is no exception. If you elect to perform "ten sets of leg extensions," you will inevitably save energy during the first nine because you have one to go. Conversely, if you restrict each effort to one set—your approach will be more aggressive. Perform one set of negative chin-ups to failure and see if you'd like to repeat a minute later. On a broader scale, your mindset during a two-hour workout differs from when you arrive twenty minutes before closing.

How long should a single exercise last?

It depends, for the most part, upon speed of movement and how many repetitions you perform. To a lesser degree it depends upon whom you ask. In the early 1970's Nautilus advocated a seven-second repetition (two seconds to lift, a one-second pause and four seconds to lower) and a repetition scheme of eight to twelve. This established time guidelines per set at fifty-six to eighty-four seconds. Research at the University of Florida in the mid 1990's revealed similar results: For the average muscle (an average mix of fast-fatigue and slow-fatigue fibers), an exercise should last between sixty and ninety seconds.

Trainer-certification groups have their own interpretation. The American College of Sports Medicine (ACSM) recommends heavy resistance and low repetitions for strength; and light-to-moderate loads and high repetitions (beyond fifteen) for muscular endurance. With one exception only, research does NOT support the contention that higher repetitions are more effective to increase muscular endurance. The ACSM has, of late, come under heavy criticism for "misrepresentation of research, lack of evidence and author bias." And they're not alone.

The National Academy of Sports Medicine (NASM) is all over the board with their proposals—one to four sets; high reps, low reps; fast speed, slow speed—feeding a warped agenda to a hungry public. And the list goes on. None of the organizations have joined the dots between strength and muscle endurance . . . which leaves everyone "up in the air," misinformed and in some cases brainwashed. Why perform a high number of repetitions when fewer repetitions produce identical strength and endurance effects?

In an extensive 2011 review of strength training research—and a subsequent article—a British team representing two major universities (Southampton Solent and Manchester Metropolitan) concluded: *"Research does not unequivocally support the superiority of a particular repetition range for enhancing any aspect of muscle function."* [2]

They believed that maintaining tension on the muscle during exercise and throughout the range of motion was a more important factor.

How long should a workout last?

The length of a workout depends on how many exercises and sets are performed. According to the same review (above), *"The vast majority of research studies show that performance of multiple sets of resistance exercise yield no greater gains than single sets performed to momentary muscular failure and therefore are not as time and energy effective."* A similar comprehensive review in 1998 found that single sets produced the same result as multiple sets in thirty-three of thirty-five studies.[3]

Despite the evidence, the one-set theory is not in common use. According to Jones, trainees are too *"willing to lend an attentive ear to 'what they want to hear,' in this case that good results can be obtained by the use of some 'easy' factor,"* easy meaning multiple sets. The common defense is, "One set is not enough." Believe what you will, the performance of one set is just as effective, more efficient, backed by research and inhibits overtraining.

Arthur Jones believed that no amount of sub-maximal training produced the same result as a single 100-percent effort in all physical endeavors. The full-out attempt forces the body to overcompensate and become stronger. He compared muscle stimulation to starting your car. Once you turn the ignition switch ON, it's ON. Further attempts waste energy and may ruin the starter. *"If you are capable of performing a second set,"* he often said, *"you didn't do the first one right."*

The recommendation of one set of twelve exercises (at sixty to ninety seconds per exercise and minimal rest between) results in a total workout time of fifteen to twenty minutes. If the workout primarily involves the use of free-weights, time will extend to thirty to forty minutes. When you can, set up free-weight stations in advance to increase the efficiency of the workout.

> **If you are capable of performing a second set, you didn't do the first one right.**

How often should you strength train?

Training frequency depends upon whom you ask. ACSM guidelines (2009) recommend that beginners train their whole body two or three times per week; intermediates three times per week (if whole body) or four (using a split routine); and advanced bodybuilders four to six times per week with split or double-split routines (twice a day—up to twenty-one hours per week). In contrast, Jones trained former Mr. Universe, Boyer Coe in 1983 twice a week for sixteen minutes (thirty-two minutes per week)—forty times less than ACSM guidelines. And he made it clear, *"If we add anything to the workout, he* (Coe) *loses size and strength almost immediately."* His records were meticulous.

The British researchers concluded the same, *"Training most major muscle groups once or twice per week is sufficient to attain strength gains equal to that of training at a greater frequency."* They found little difference between one, two or three times per week with trained or untrained individuals.

There are two types of "fatigue" associated with resistance training: one, muscular; the other, systemic. The first is local; the second, global . . . and the two are related. Every exercise produces fatigue at the local level AND, to a lesser degree, the global level. The greater the size of the muscle, the quantity of muscle involved in the exercise or the intensity of effort, the greater the effect on the system. The difference is similar to that encountered by throwing a large versus small rock into a body of water. The large rock makes a bigger splash and propels a higher wave across the surface. Large waves in exercise increase recovery time and increased recovery time means less-frequent stimulation . . .

. . . with one exception. Advanced trainees believe they are immune to fatigue and their apparent success leads others to believe that they MUST be right. At fourteen I was fortunate that I did *not* have the means to "lift weights" in a public facility. Fortunate, because the guy with the biggest arms would have held me spellbound. I would have copied his style and if I was bold enough to ask, he would have anointed me with his great wisdom. And fortunate that Jones arrived to save the day:

"If you are training in a gym with the current Mr. America," he said, *"and if you like him personally, you will rather naturally look upon his advice*

as sound, 'after all, he did win, didn't he?'—but in fact, with his potential, perhaps he should have won earlier—maybe his own firmly held beliefs have delayed his progress enormously." [4]

He added . . .

"Most well-known bodybuilders have followed so many different routines by the time they finally do attain a point of recognition that they really have no slightest idea regarding "which routine produced which result"—but they almost invariably think they do; which is, I suppose, another natural mistake—but a mistake, nevertheless."

And concluded . . .

"It's a shame that bodybuilding is wasted on bodybuilders."

Advanced trainees generally address "recovery" by disassociating local and global fatigue. As a result, they train their body in parts—today legs, tomorrow chest and back, next day biceps and shoulders—endless combinations. Their rationale is simple: If they work their biceps into submission on Friday and don't get around to them again until next Thursday, they will have five days of "rest." But the biceps aren't "at rest" when ONE, they are used in upper-back exercises Monday; TWO, lug weight plates around the gym Tuesday; THREE, are anatomically adjacent to working muscles Wednesday; and FOUR, attached to the body when *any* muscle is worked. The body is a whole, and local work affects the whole. A muscle may recover from exercise but the system must also recover so that it can favorably respond to the next stimulation. Conversely, the system may recover from a workout while a muscle has not. If either (system or muscle) is NOT ready for the next signal, the response will not be the one you desire.

The purpose of exercise is to stimulate change—and the body responds in one of three ways: maintenance, growth or decline. The choice it makes is often related to training frequency.

I watched a gym owner from Gainesville, Florida, perform four repetitions on a MedX Lumbar Extension machine during a demonstration in Ocala in the late 1980's. According to Arthur Jones who had measured the subject's adaptive ability on more than 100 occasions, it would take his lumbar muscles approximately two and a half weeks to recover from thirty seconds of exercise. The subject possessed an unusually high percentage of fast-twitch muscle fibers which made fatigue eminent and recovery difficult. The man looked and "felt" fine days later, but his muscles were far from recovered:

"When a muscle has been worked to a point of momentary failure by heavy exercise, the situation is just that—the muscle has "failed MOMENTARILY." But in most cases, within three seconds—or less—the muscle has recovered approximately fifty percent of the strength it had lost as a result of the exercise; but it does not follow that it will then be fully recovered in six seconds, or even six minutes—full recovery usually takes MORE THAN twenty-four hours, frequently as much as forty to sixty hours. But even if the muscle itself does recover entirely, this is no indication that the system—which supplies the muscle—is fully recovered." [5]

To look and "feel" fine is not enough—yet, tools to measure the recovery phenomenon are rare. There is no dipstick to declare readiness for the next effort. The only tool you have is a workout chart. Check numbers. If you have good form, high intensity and still lack progress, perform fewer exercises with less frequency so your system can properly recover. The advice is more applicable to those advanced: *"An advanced trainee does NOT need 'more' exercise than a beginner; he simply needs 'harder' exercise, in direct proportion to the differential in strength. An advanced man may be able to 'stand' more exercise—but it is not a requirement, and will almost always quickly lead to a situation where additional progress comes to a halt, or slows to a snail's pace."* [6]

Ellington Darden described it his way. *"As you get stronger, you must do less overall exercise to continue to get even stronger. The reason goes back to that thing called recovery ability. Your recovery ability does not increase in proportion to your ability to get stronger."* [7]

> **Instead of trying to determine how much exercise we can tolerate, perhaps we should try to determine how little we actually require.**

Suggestions from his 2004 book, *The New High Intensity Training* follow:

Start with three sessions per week. When progress stalls, reduce workout frequency to two hard and one easy workout per week—"easy" defined as stopping two repetitions short of muscle failure during the middle workout of the week. When progress stalls again, regress to two workouts per week. At the same time, gradually reduce the number of exercises in each workout from twelve to ten to eight. The entire process (as described in this paragraph) may take twelve months. Chart you workouts meticulously and when in doubt, perform *less* exercise.

The major premise of high-intensity exercise was written anonymously more than ninety years ago: *"Instead of trying to determine how much exercise we can tolerate, perhaps we should try to determine how little we actually require."*

REFERENCES

[1] Jones, A., *Nautilus Training Principles Bulletin No. 2*, 22: 61, 1971.

[2] Fisher, J., Steele, J., Bruce-Low, S., Smith, D., "Evidence-Based Resistance Training Recommendations," *Medicina Sportiva*, Med Sport 15 (3): 147-162, 2011.

[3] Carpinelli, R.N., Otto, R.M., "Strength Training: Single Versus Multiple Sets," *Sports Med*; 26: 73-84, 1998.

[4] Jones, A., *Nautilus Training Principles Bulletin No. 2*, 32: 91, 1971.

[5] Jones, A., *Nautilus Training Principles Bulletin No. 2*, 21: 57, 1971.

[6] Jones, A., *Nautilus Training Principles Bulletin No. 2*, 6: 19, 1971.

[7] Darden, E., Ph.D., *The New High Intensity Training*, Rodale, Inc., 11: 89, 2004.

CHAPTER 6

···

Exercise Form and Speed of Movement

"As I look back on my 45 years of bodybuilding experience, combined with thousands and thousands of individuals I've trained (and observed training), I can say with confidence that more people would profit from an understanding and application of proper form, than from proper intensity. Of course, in the long run, you're going to need large amounts of both."

Ellington Darden, Ph.D.

As I look back I can likewise say with confidence that the greatest legacy a trainer can leave is to enter every exercise facility in the country and holler two words with a bull-horn: "SLOW DOWN." People lift weights too quickly and men are more at fault than women. In my facility I controlled form and intensity by having every workout of every client supervised, which did not guarantee quality. Labor was cheap and I retained a saying: "If you want to learn how to properly use a piece of equipment, watch a woman, not a man." It's as true today as then—and I won't touch it with a ten-foot pole.

Without a single *other* modification, a reduced speed of movement during progressive resistance exercise would probably double the results of current trainees.

The message has eluded most:

- Some won't listen—usually Type A's who insist on doing things their way. I wish I had the money to waste.
- Slow makes exercise hard. Most trainees don't want hard; they want exercise. "Hard" takes them out of their comfort zone and spawns a surplus of excuses.
- The human body doesn't like hard. When hard appears, it seeks easy—like moving more quickly during exercise.
- Many believe that "fast" is better than "slow," especially when training for explosive sports.

In June of 2012, I watched a Golf Channel® presentation on the preparation of PGA Tour professionals. One trainer stated: *"Golf is an explosive sport, so you have to train that way."* To make his point he had his client jump from the floor to a thigh-high box and down—sometimes with two legs, sometimes with one. If Arthur Jones had been on the set, he would have drawn a pistol and put the lad away. One useless concept after another provided an hour of comic relief.

Led by the famous TPI (Titleist Performance Institute®) program, golfers have been brainwashed into thinking that they need something special, and worse, that the need is being addressed by the sports/medical group overseeing the fitness vans and by functional specialists at the public end. It is refreshing to see a growing concern for fitness in golf (I never thought I'd see it in my lifetime), but alarming to see the direction in which game is being led—far from where it should be, which leaves the athletes far from where they could be.

In most cases bad form is inseparable from speed of movement, but it's not the entire story. Good form begins with proper execution of each and every repetition, as described:

"A properly performed repetition should proceed as follows:

- *Assume a safe and productive position from which to work.*
- *Grasp the bar or handle, or contact the pad of the movement-arm (machine).*

🔊 *SLOWLY apply force against the bar, movement-arm or pad until it begins to move. Maintain a constant pressure on the resistance so that it continues to move SLOWLY, without momentum, to the end of the range of motion. Feel the weight being lifted every inch of the way. When the resistance reaches the end of the range (a theoretical position of complete contraction), do ONE of the following TO KEEP TENSION ON THE MUSCLE:*

    1. *If it is difficult to hold the weight in that position, pause for a second or two.*

    2. *If it is easy to hold the weight there, don't pause or fully extend your limbs. Exercises that push away from the body's center, such as chest, leg and shoulder presses, dips and squats, fall in this category. If it is difficult to distinguish, close your eyes and hold an extended pause. It won't take long to find out.*

🔊 *After the pause/no-pause scenario, reduce the applied force and allow the weight to return SLOWLY to its original position without touching the weight stack.*

🔊 *Repeat a smooth, controlled lifting and lowering exertion until the weight no longer moves using an all-out effort (and without throwing or jerking)." [1]*

To that I'll add:

🔊 If the exercise station has a seat belt or mechanism to secure your position, USE IT to better isolate the movement and diminish the contribution of other muscles.

🔊 Relax all body parts *not* involved in the exercise. This takes a conscious effort especially during the final repetitions. The best opportunity to relax presents itself when muscles are lowering weight. A glance at the weight stack should help.

🔊 Do not grip handles tightly for a prolonged time during exercise as it elevates blood pressure to high and dangerous levels. If you must grip tightly during the lifting phase or to pause in a contracted position (as during leg extensions), relax during the lowering phase.

🔊 Do not "make faces" during exercise. Muscle contraction triggers the distribution of blood to areas of perceived need. When you exercise legs, you don't want blood directed to arms. The neck and shoulder area is particularly vulnerable to tension during upper-body exercise. If your neck gets tight, move it around without interrupting the effort.

- Don't hold your breath for a prolonged time during exercise. Oxygen to the working muscles is vital but it doesn't matter how it gets there. Some trainers advocate a pattern—exhale during the lifting phase and inhale during the lowering phase. While that may suffice during the early repetitions of a set, it proves inadequate during the final efforts when eight to ten breaths *per repetition* may be required. Breathe as needed and don't hold your breath.
- Speed of motion is critical to form and, as Jones suggests, *"Without good form, there is little or nothing of value left in exercise."* To control your pace, try one of the following:

1. Time a pre-determined cadence (two seconds up; four seconds down—as a minimum)
2. Time yourself for eight to twelve repetitions to ensure that speed remains less than six to eight seconds per effort. Consider that the range of motion of some exercises is greater than others.
3. Train by "feel." Use a pace that allows you to "feel" the resistance, with no momentum, every inch of the way. It may help to close your eyes.
4. Once in a while don't count repetitions. Perform each exercise at a fraction of your normal speed and continue until nothing moves.
5. If you believe the exercise you are performing will easily exceed twelve repetitions, ask yourself at nine or ten, "How slow can I go and still make it?" and on the next, "How slow can I *now* go and still make it?" and on the next . . .
6. Stand in front of a clock with a large second hand. "Lift in ten seconds, lower in five and DON'T take your eyes off the clock." Use a weight that allows the performance of ten repetitions and hope that you make five. Slow can be a humbling experience.

Without good form, there is little or nothing of value left in exercise.

No one has discovered an *ideal* cadence for strength training. Slow is definitely harder than fast but how slow is best? A definition began with the introduction of "Super Slow" and the modification of equipment to better suit the needs of a slow cadence—ten seconds to lift, five or ten to lower. The Center for Exercise Science at the University of Florida took it a step beyond by conducting a study in which only two repetitions per exercise were performed: The first, twenty seconds up, a twenty-second hold in the contracted position and twenty seconds down; the second, ten seconds up, a ten-second hold and ten seconds down. If you completed the full ninety seconds in good form, resistance was increased by 5% during the next workout. The results trumped that of traditional training.

Despite ongoing efforts to identify an ideal cadence, the following has been established: A slower speed of movement during exercise is safer, more productive and more likely to result in good form. And that, according to Arthur Jones, is a good thing: *"In exercise as in most things,"* he said, *"form (or style of performance) may not be the only thing, but it is certainly a prerequisite for good results."* [2]

The potential for speed during exercise is dictated by the amount of resistance used relative to the existing level of strength. You cannot lift heavy weights rapidly: You *must* throw them to move them—and doing so will not build strength . . .

. . . but it will do other things:

". . . a fast speed of movement during exercise does the following: it jerks the muscle violently during the first few degrees of movement . . . after which point the weight is moving so fast that the muscles literally are not involved in the rest of the movement. The result being that a dangerous yank is imposed on the muscles at the start of the movement then absolutely nothing is accomplished during most of the movement. In such cases you are throwing the weight not lifting it . . . and such a style of training will produce nothing but injuries." [3]

The Nautilus inventor routinely demonstrated the forces involved during exercise by connecting a force plate (a platform that resembled an oversized bathroom scale) to a large oscilloscope so that his audience could see first-hand the effect of speed on exercise. The presentations I witnessed featured MedX general manager, Jim Flanagan who mounted the plate with a sixty-pound barbell in hand. At 6'5" and 260 pounds, Jim started moving the weight slowly from his shoulders to overhead and back. At a slow speed the resistance remained close to its value—fifty-eight to sixty-two pounds. Jim steadily increased his speed, eventually slamming the weight up and down above his head. The once-smooth wave on the oscilloscope left the screen, top and bottom. At the moment the barbell was jerked (with Jim's hands at shoulder height), the force exceeded 200 pounds, more than three times its weight. From there the barbell weighed less than zero for most of its remaining voyage. The resistance was lifting Jim's arms, instead of the opposite. Loud and clear, LIFTING WEIGHTS RAPIDLY IS NEITHER PRODUCTIVE NOR SAFE.

The charts below (Figures 1 and 2) provide a visual comparison of the variance of resistance that occurs during "slow" versus "fast" speeds.

Figure 1: **SLOW MOVEMENT SPEED DURING EXERCISE**

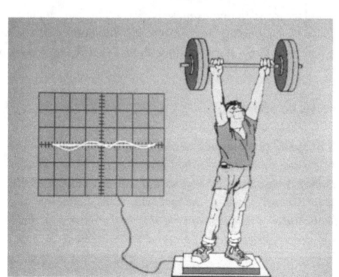

Figure 2: **FAST MOVEMENT SPEED DURING EXERCISE**

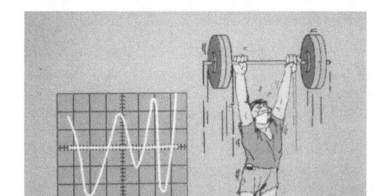

Effort increases during exercise from repetition to repetition. As fatigue sets in, the final repetitions demand the greatest input. Despite that, the speed of movement should remain about the same throughout, until of course, momentary failure grinds it to a halt. Speed should be slow and controlled during the first few repetitions (for safety), and slow and controlled toward the final efforts due to fatigue. In the real world most trainees "panic" during the final repetitions which causes speed to increase. Look for the signs: At the end of a set, effort will increase by necessity but speed should decrease. Always perform as many repetitions as possible in good form.

What do the experts say about speed? The American College of Sports Medicine recommends what they call variable "repetition durations" for strength. Untrained individuals are encouraged to move at slow-to-moderate velocities while trained individuals are allowed the freedom of a continuum from slow to fast. Why the difference? No explanation. The ACSM also believes that fast, explosive movements improve sports performance, notably vertical jump and sprint times. *"Fast velocities,"* they say, *"have been shown to be more effective for enhanced muscular performance capacities (e.g. number of repetitions performed, work and power output, and volume)."* While it is obvious that more repetitions can be performed at increased speeds, their vague statement fails to address what training methods "best" stimulate physiological enhancement. It also fails to identify the "dangers" associated with fast-velocity training.

And it lacks credibility. A recent mega-review of literature related to strength-training methodology concluded: *"Comprehensive reviews of this area of research have reported that resistance training at shorter repetition durations* (faster speeds) *produced no greater strength or power increases than training at longer repetition durations* (slower speeds)." [4] One of the studies cited by the review team was their own. It concluded: *"There was no evidence to suggest that these techniques* (Olympic lifting and plyometric exercises, both of which advocate explosive movements) *can enhance strength and/or sporting performance (including vertical jump and sprint) to any greater degree than traditional weight training methods."* [5]

Arthur Jones summed up his take on speed of movement during exercise: *"It is easily possible to move too fast during exercise, but probably impossible to move too slowly; that says it all, everything that needs to be said."* [6]

In spite of the facts, trainers are knocking down the door to get certified by the ACSM. Pray you don't get one.

It is easily possible to move too fast during exercise, but probably impossible to move too slowly; that says it all, everything that needs to be said.

REFERENCES

[1] Bannister, G., "The Repetition," *In Arthur's Shadow*, Cork Hill Press, Jan. 8:13, 2005.

[2] Jones, A., "Negative Accentuated Strength Training," Peterson, J.A. Ph.D. (editor), *Total Fitness the Nautilus Way*, Leisure Press, 10: 106, 1978.

[3] Jones, A., "Avoiding and Preventing injuries," Peterson, J.A. Ph.D. (editor), *Total Fitness the Nautilus Way*, Leisure Press, 6: 69, 1978.

[4] Fisher, J., Steele, J., Bruce-Low, S., Smith, D., "Evidence-Based Resistance Training Recommendations," Medicina Sportiva, Med Sport 15 (3): 147-162, 2011.

[5] Bruce-Low, S., Smith, D., "Explosive Exercise in Sports Training: A Critical Review," *Journal of Exercise Physiology 2007*; 10; 21-33.

[6] Jones, A., *The Lumbar Spine*, Sequoia Communications, 1988.

CHAPTER 7

....

Number of Repetitions

How many repetitions should you perform? Some research studies have identified low (three to six) and high (fifteen to twenty) repetition ranges but the majority single out a range of eight to twelve for best results from strength training. Despite that, many trainees adopt personal preferences by trial and error.

In January of 1986 Arthur Jones introduced science to the question by developing a computerized medical Leg Extension machine that measured the immediate *effect* of exercise. After testing a large number of subjects he believed that *inroad* (defined as *"the depletion of momentary strength from a set of exercise"*) was an important factor in growth stimulation. Specifically, he discovered that an inroad of 20-25% stimulated the most efficient rate of muscular growth for all major muscle structures. That is, the number of repetitions performed should reduce a muscle's starting strength by 20-25%. The new device could easily determine the *exact* repetition at which that occurred.

From early experience Jones was aware of a relationship between muscle strength and local muscular endurance:

When I was able, but barely able, to lift 100 pounds only once, then I knew that I could perform exactly 10 repetitions with 83 pounds . . . no more, no less, not nine, not eleven, exactly ten.

When I was able to perform ten repetitions with 100 pounds, then I knew that I could perform one repetition with exactly 120.

When my strength changed, up or down, my anaerobic (local muscular) endurance went up or down to exactly the same degree.

Thus, when I reached a point of momentary muscular failure, after having performed exactly ten repetitions with 83 percent of my starting level of positive strength . . . then, at that point in the exercise, I failed because my remaining strength was slightly below 83 percent of my starting level.

So, ten repetitions with 83 percent of my starting strength level reduced my strength momentarily, by about 18 percent.

Being clearly aware of this ratio in myself, I assumed that it applied to other people as well . . . thus, when I encountered a man who could perform only four repetitions with 80 percent of his starting level, I first accused him of not trying hard enough.

But he was trying, although I failed to recognize this at the time; that was all he could do; his ratio was different.

Later, another man performed twenty-three repetitions with 80 percent of his starting strength level, and again I was surprised.

These and other examples finally made me aware of the fact that this ratio varies on an individual basis . . . but I simply overlooked what should have been the obvious implications.

For years, many more years than I even like to remember, I have been telling people to train in much the same way; select a weight, by trial and error, that will permit you to perform seven or eight repetitions in good form; but continue for as many repetitions as you can in good form, stopping only when it becomes momentarily impossible to continue.

Then, during later workouts, always perform as many repetitions as possible . . . but when it becomes possible to perform ten or more repetitions in good form, then increase the weight about 5 percent. Never use a weight that will not permit at least seven repetitions, and always increase the weight slightly when it becomes possible to perform ten or more repetitions.

Most other people have been giving very similar advice for the last fifty years . . . and millions of people have trained in this manner.

But I now understand that this advice is wrong . . . wrong for many people; and I understand why it is wrong.[1]

According to Ellington Darden who was present when Jones introduced the computerized testing device, approximately 70% of trainees produced good results from a repetition range of eight to twelve. Further tests on an advanced version of the tool established that seventy-two percent (72%) of subjects fatigued at a rate of 2% per repetition. Twenty-eight percent (28%) fatigued at faster or slower rates and, therefore, did not respond as favorably to the prescribed repetition range of eight to twelve.

The following charts represent computer printouts of two subjects who exerted maximum force during each repetition of a test on Jones' original Leg Extension device. The 75% line (on both charts) signified where the ideal inroad of 25% occurred. Figure 1 demonstrates a subject who performed only three repetitions before his strength level fell below 75% of his first-repetition strength (represented as 100%). By contrast, the subject in Figure 2 required seventeen repetitions before he fell below 75% of his starting strength—required 5.67 times as many repetitions to create an inroad similar to that of the subject in Figure 1 (inroads of 27% and 30% respectively).

The determination of an ideal number of repetitions demands the creation of an inroad sufficient to stimulate, but not too great to prevent growth. The subject in Figure 1 required few repetitions to reach an ideal inroad while the subject in Figure 2 required a greater number. A range of eight to twelve, as generally recommended, would probably create recovery issues for the subject in Figure 1 but fail to stimulate the subject in Figure 2.

Figure 1: Subject 599

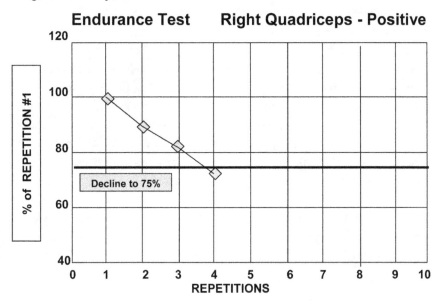

Figure 2: Subject 290

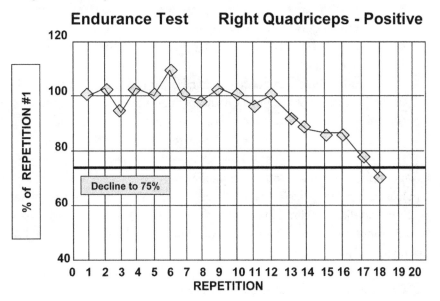

The above examples were not "extreme." Following several hundred tests (in 1987), one subject performed only one repetition with 80% of his maximum strength while another performed thirty-four repetitions with more than 80% of his maximum. In later tests one subject could not perform one repetition with any weight that represented more than 50% of his maximum, while others *gained* strength following hundreds of repetitions. Jones called the phenomenon "neurological efficiency." Muscles that display rapid fatigue possess an abundance of fast-twitch (strong, powerful) fibers, while those that fatigue at a slow rate possess an abundance of slow-twitch (endurance) fibers. And there's nothing you can do about it. According to Darden, *"All reports indicate that neurological efficiency is genetic and not subject to modification through training."* [2]

The intriguing discoveries were made with equipment rarely available to the public. But there is good news: Common equipment (barbells or machines) and the following guidelines can be used to establish "ideal" repetition schemes:

1. Determine your one-repetition maximum weight on any exercise.*(read the **Caution** below)
2. Rest at least five minutes.
3. Using 80% of that maximum, perform as many repetitions as possible in good form (without cheating). Note the number.
4. Multiply that number by .15 and round the result to the nearest whole number.
5. Add the whole number to the number of repetitions performed in step #3 to establish the high end of your ideal repetition range.
6. Subtract the whole number from the repetitions performed in step #3 to establish the low end of your range.

For example, if your one-repetition maximum (how much you can lift one time) on a leg-curl machine is 150 pounds and you later perform a set of eight repetitions with 120 pounds (150 x 80%) in good form, your "ideal" repetition scheme would be calculated as follows: 8 x .15 = 1.2 (rounded to 1)

8 repetitions + 1 = 9 (the high end of the range)
8 repetitions - 1 = 7 (the low end of the range)

In this case, best results from the leg-curl machine would be produced by seven to nine repetitions of exercise. The performance of less than seven indicates a weight too high; nine or more should trigger an increase in weight during the next workout.

*Caution: The test to determine how much you can lift one time is dangerous. The trial-and-error process exposes muscles and joint systems to high forces. Proceed with caution and use spotters.

Dr. Darden made several observations during the practical application of the test (above):

- In general, trainees required higher-than-guideline repetitions on the leg press because of the use of multiple muscles and joints and because of the inherent "rest" encountered near full extension.

- Trainees often performed more repetitions during free-weight work than with similar machine exercise (Hammer, Nautilus, etc.). Free-weights do not work muscles as thoroughly through a range of motion as machines and, in some positions, offer a "rest."

- It was *not* necessary to test all muscle groups. Trainees generally tested the same (or close to the same) in all lower-body exercises, exhibited a unique fatigue pattern throughout upper-body torso muscles and a discrete pattern with the muscles of the arms. As such, one test can be performed in each of three areas—lower-body, upper-body and arms—and results applied to *all* exercises in that area.

- Multi-joint exercise tests are not as accurate as single-joint tests for obvious reasons. The involvement of numerous muscles with unique fatigue characteristics could create a hybrid repetition scheme ideal to none.

- Speed of movement is important. The performance of twelve repetitions in fifteen seconds differs from the same in ninety seconds. Many exercise physiologists believe that the optimal chemical process within the muscle occurs when exercise duration is thirty to ninety seconds. They recommend: sixty seconds for a muscle with an average mix of fibers, thirty to forty seconds for a predominance of fast-twitch fibers and eighty to ninety seconds for a muscle with a predominance of slow-twitch fibers. Jones used a speed of six seconds per repetition (three up, three down) during his 1986 testing. He recorded—but did not focus on—total time. In any case, with 70% of subjects performing eight to twelve repetitions using 80% of their one-repetition maximum, the total training time remained within the parameters of physiological research: forty-eight to seventy-two seconds.

If you opt not to perform a one-repetition maximum strength test, use eight to twelve repetitions on all exercises for a month. Stay with it as long as your strength increases by 5% every two weeks. If progress is less, test using two exercises—the leg extension and standing barbell curl. Use the results of the leg extension test for all lower-body exercises and the results of the biceps test for all upper-body exercises. Multi-joint tests are not reliable by nature: Use eight to twelve repetitions on *all* compound movements.

REFERENCES

[1] Jones, A., "Exercise . . . '86: The Present State of the Art," The Arthur Jones Collection, Bodyworx Publishing: 1227.

[2] Darden, E., Ph.D., *Massive Muscles in 10 Weeks*, 1987.

CHAPTER 8

....

The Importance
of Full-Range Exercise

T he creation of tools that isolated muscle function and accurately measured strength through a full range of motion spawned a new era of research that spread from the front porch of a home in Florida to the exercise physiology labs of several prominent universities: The University of Florida, The University of California, San Diego and Syracuse University. The years were 1972-1986. The porch belonged to Arthur Jones.

As was his style he called the breakthrough, *"The most significant discovery in the history of exercise . . . a discovery that will send shock waves around the world, a discovery that will change exercise forever, and change it for the better."* It did.

The tools could measure both the "effect" (immediate, short-term consequence) and the "results" (long-term benefits) of exercise. A three-part procedure was used to determine the "effect" of exercise on the muscle's starting strength:

- A test of "fresh" strength.
- An exercise performed on the same machine and continued to momentary muscle failure.
- A test of "exhausted" strength IMMEDIATELY after the exercise.

The results revealed a range of responses as reported in the previous chapter. Some trainees fatigued after a few repetitions, while others demonstrated an *increase* in strength on the post-exercise test.

Jones paraded two subjects who demonstrated extreme responses around the country—and was forced to re-think his "one-shoe-fits-all" approach. But thinking was his nature and he soon devised a hybrid test. If full-range exercise had an immediate "effect" on the muscle (as observed), what would be the "effect" of performing a partial-range exercise? The three-part procedure evolved:

- A test of full-range "fresh" strength.
- A partial range-of-motion exercise continued to momentary muscle failure.
- A test of full-range "exhausted" strength IMMEDIATELY after the exercise.

The charts that follow (Figures 1 and 2) demonstrate the test results of two subjects on the MedX Medical Leg Extension machine:

Figure 1: **RESPONSE TO EXERCISE - TYPE S**

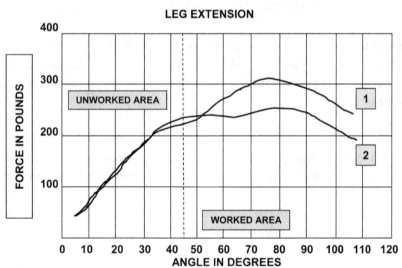

Figure 1 shows two curves that represent tests taken less than six minutes apart to determine the strength of the muscles of the front thigh. The top curve (#1) represents the PRE-exercise test; the bottom curve (#2), the POST-exercise test. The exercise (between tests) was performed with both legs and continued to momentary failure using a resistance based on the subject's starting strength (one that would allow approximately ten repetitions)—but it was NOT full-range. The exercise was restricted to the first half of the movement (from the starting position to approximately halfway up, represented by the right side of the chart and identified as WORKED AREA). As can be seen, the "effect" (immediate consequence) of the exercise was limited to the WORKED AREA. Little to no fatigue occurred on the left side of the chart where the subject performed no work. Jones classified the "effect" as "TYPE-S," a SPECIFIC response to exercise—fatigue where you work; no fatigue where you don't—exactly what you'd expect. Further tests revealed other characteristics of TYPE-S subjects:

- The "effect" was similar in magnitude when exercise was restricted to the last half of the movement (left side of chart).
- Prolonged partial-range exercise produced "results" that mirrored the "effect." TYPE-S subjects produced long-term results ONLY where they worked, and little to none where they did not.
- Approximately 72% of a random group showed a TYPE-S response to exercise.

Figure 2: **RESPONSE TO EXERCISE - TYPE G**

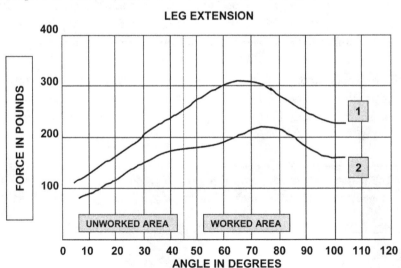

Figure 2 shows two curves that represent the same test procedure as Figure 1. The response from this subject was unique and led Jones to believe that he did not cooperate or that there was an error. Work performed on the right side of the chart ONLY produced a proportionate effect throughout the range of motion. The muscle fatigued equally where work was performed AND where NO work was performed. Jones classified this "effect" as "TYPE-G," a GENERAL response to exercise—fatigue where you work; fatigue where you don't—not what you'd expect.

The test characteristics of TYPE-G subjects follow:

- The "effect" was similar in magnitude when exercise was restricted to the last half of the movement (left side of chart).
- The response was similar with long-term exercise. TYPE-G subjects produced full-range "results" from the performance of partial-range exercise, regardless of where exercise was performed.
- Approximately 28% of a random group showed a TYPE-G response to exercise.

The same phenomenon surfaced with tests conducted on the MedX Lumbar Extension machine. Approximately 80% of a random group of subjects tested as TYPE-S, while 20% were TYPE-G. The percentage of TYPE-S and TYPE-G subjects varied from muscle to muscle but established a trend: The majority of trainees exhibit a TYPE-S response to exercise. They fatigue and produce results ONLY in the range of motion where exercise occurs.

Following thousands of tests on untrained subjects, Jones compared the average strength curve of a TYPE-S and TYPE-G subject to the ideal strength curve on the Lumbar Extension (Figure 3) and Leg Extension machines (Figure 4), below:

> **The majority of trainees exhibit a TYPE-S response to exercise: They fatigue and produce results ONLY in the range of motion where exercise occurs.**

Figure 3:

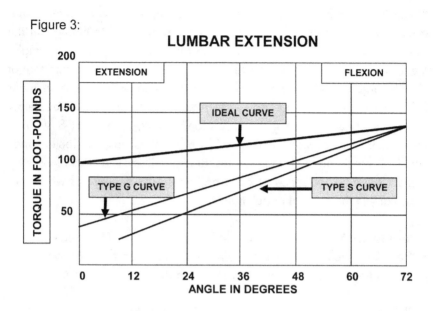

Figure 4:

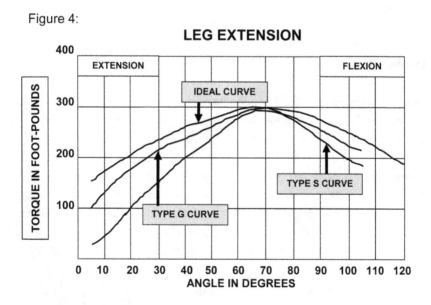

The "ideal curve" in both charts represents the distribution of resistance to the muscle provided by the machine's cam during exercise AND the shape a curve will ultimately take when strength is proportionate throughout the range of motion—when the muscle is as strong as it can be at every angle, the IDEAL. In both charts the curve of TYPE-G subjects is flatter than that of TYPE-S subjects and generally stronger in the weakest test position (near full extension, left side of chart). Nonetheless, both curves are well below "ideal" levels of strength in full extension. In fact, many TYPE-S subjects tested on the lumbar machine (Figure 3) were so weak in extension that they could not reach the final angles to test at all, as illustrated. This alone may explain the high incidence of back problems—the majority of which are muscular—in the general population.

Jones suspected that the strength difference favoring TYPE-G subjects was a *"carry-over from the normal activities that produced their strength in the peak position . . . a carry-over that TYPE-S individuals do not get."*

TYPE-S individuals benefit from exercise ONLY in the range in which they work. TYPE-G individuals receive full-range benefits from partial-range exercise. The implications are clear.

Implications

Most muscles have TYPE-S tendencies: They require full-range resistance to develop full-range strength—the quest for which begins and ends with equipment.

Today's trends have led many to believe that barbells and machines are non-functional. As a result, trainees have been lured to seek other sources of resistance: bodyweight, latex bands, pulleys or gimmicks that show up in the training environment. Most are fine if you have nothing else, but they fail to deliver a resistance that meets the needs of a working muscle throughout

---

In fact, many TYPE-S subjects tested on the lumbar machine were so weak in extension that they could not reach the final angles to test at all.

---

a full-range movement and fail to provide an adequate stimulus for growth. There are better choices.

The most common tool, the barbell, fails for the same reason. Gravity pulls straight down while body parts rotate around an axis. The difference results in leverage changes—some favorable, some not—that affect the delivery of resistance to the muscle. The difference led Arthur Jones to develop a tool that delivered "full-range exercise."

The following chart, Figure 5, compares the application of resistance to the upper-arm during a biceps curl with a barbell versus a Nautilus machine.

Figure 5:

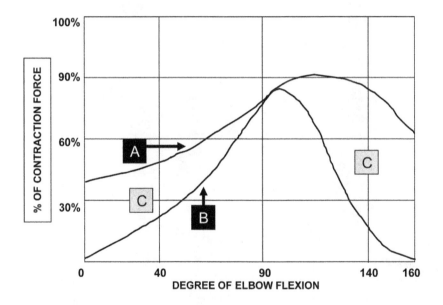

BARBELL versus NAUTILUS® CURL

The top curve (A) represents the ideal strength curve of a biceps curl performed on a Nautilus machine (dictated by output and provided by the machine's cam). The bottom curve (B) depicts the actual resistance provided by a barbell during a biceps curl. The area between the curves (C) shows the difference between real and ideal, the additional benefit provided by the use of a machine with a proper cam.

Not all machines deliver resistance to the muscles as they should. But, if the cam is proper and the machine "delivers as advertized," it provides a constant challenge to the working muscles every inch of the way—a challenge that must be "felt" to be appreciated.

One trainee's description of that difference (C, above) may help explain the current trend in exercise: *"A bench press with a barbell will get your attention; a chest press on a Nautilus machine will wipe you out."*

Where and when possible, select an exercise tool that provides an adequate resistance over as great a range of motion as possible. With the majority of trainees, full-range strength requires the application of full-range resistance.

CHAPTER 9

●●

Equipment

Anything that makes exercise harder makes it more productive.

One thing was apparent: Arthur Jones was intrigued by "anything and everything" that made exercise more demanding.

In that accord he wrote the following: *"The four steps of meaningful progression in the field of physical training have been (1) calisthenics, (2) gymnastics, (3) weight training and (4) Nautilus training . . . The various steps have each provided a marked increase in the degree of possible results, and simultaneously a reduction in the required amount of training . . . both provided by the same factor in all cases—each step produced a marked increase in the possible 'intensity of effort;' gymnastics are harder than calisthenics—weight-training is harder than gymnastics—and Nautilus training is harder than conventional weight-training . . . From the very start of the investigations that finally produced the Nautilus methods and systems of training we were clearly aware of 'what was needed'—HARDER EXERCISE."* [1]

The quality of resistance made each step progressive. Calisthenics used part of your bodyweight; gymnastics used it all. Weight-training added resistance to bodyweight or to the weight of body parts, while Nautilus training improved the quality and delivery of resistance to the working muscles.

The act of lifting weight against gravity involves muscular input. The pull of gravity is vertical—straight down, which makes the vertical portion—and

ONLY the vertical portion of an exercise movement—the toughest and most productive.

It's harder to lift your car than push it.

Joint systems, however, move rotationally—and that doesn't mix well with the pull of gravity. Leverage changes with *every* angle of movement during exercise which is why bodyweight and free-weight resistance "feels" different in every position. At some angles the leverage change results in a "sticking point" where the weight feels relatively *heavy*; at others, a "lock-out" where NO resistance is apparent. Another point: The only position in which a muscle can activate as many fibers as possible (for the purpose of force production and strength gain) is full-contraction—a position where most free-weight and bodyweight exercises provide little-to-no resistance. Therefore, because of the random change of resistance and the considerable variation in available strength during movement, neither free-weights nor bodyweight can provide full-range exercise.

You can't negotiate a curve in the road by driving in a straight line.

For more than twenty-two years, Jones sought to negotiate the curve by driving around it. In the process he identified the ingredients that comprised what he called "a perfect form of exercise."

- **Positive Work**. Almost all forms of exercise provide positive work—lifting a weight. But positive-only work (the core of isokinetic training) lacks several ingredients of productive exercise.
- **Negative Work Potential.** The provision of negative work—the "back force" that opposes the direction of pull during exercise—was necessary at all angles to produce optimal strength and flexibility. Many traditional exercises fail to provide a "back force" in key positions.
- **Direct Resistance**. The direct application of resistance to the working muscles through the use of pads ensured that the muscle targeted would be the first to fatigue.
- **Variable Resistance**. Resistance had to match the strength potential of the muscle as it moved. The automatic variation was

ultimately provided by an elliptical cam that shared a common axis with the moving parts.

- **Rotary-Form Resistance**. A resistance that matched the rotational nature of the human joint system (as opposed to the straight-line or gravitational resistance provided by traditional tools).
- **Balanced Resistance**. The movement arms of the new tools required a "counterbalance" to preserve the integrity of the resistance throughout the movement. Exercise without counter-weighting resulted in extreme and dangerous fluctuations in the applied weight.
- **Full-Range Resistance**. Resistance had to challenge a muscle through a full range of motion to stimulate full-range strength. With few exceptions, free-weight and pulley-station exercises fail to provide adequate resistance in a position of full contraction.
- **Omni-Directional Resistance.** The application of straight-line resistance to rotary movement is appropriate and effective at only ONE angle—the angle at which the pull of the muscle directly opposes that of the resistance. A proper cam assured that this requirement was met at EVERY angle, regardless of the direction of pull.
- **Unrestricted Speed of Movement.** The ability to move as quickly or as slowly as desired. At the time, some forms of exercise (namely isokinetics) featured a constant speed of movement during training and testing—a method that proved dangerous, ineffective and inaccurate.

Jones incorporated all of the ingredients into tools that made exercise more demanding—but success was an uphill climb.

Bodybuilding at the time was controlled by Joe Weider who immediately launched a series of attacks to discredit "anything Jones" through his magazine empire and panel of experts—doctors, physiologists, fitness gurus and bodybuilders. His audience trusted the source and Weider's high-volume training philosophy and free-weight bias prevailed. And where it did not, it stirred great debate. To this day bodybuilders believe that nothing can replace a barbell—as if they know how to use a barbell.

Case in point: Two orthopedic surgeons from Caracas were introduced to Nautilus machines in New York City around the time I arrived in Venezuela. The trainer probably salivated when the pair of twenty-year bodybuilders entered his domain. From all reports, he "killed them with a hard workout." The surgeons took a stance. They concurred that the cam specific to each machine unduly stressed tendons when the muscle reached a stretched position, that the lack of a "sticking point" during exercise meant something was wrong and that the machines were somehow dangerous. The observations were not unusual for trainees with a free-weight background. The machines *were* different and the two *were* perceptive. "Sticking points" *are* eliminated by a device that automatically adjusts resistance to match available strength—strength they both lacked in full extension.

The pair also disapproved of the method. When I hosted them in my facility two years later, they rejected muscle failure, refused to move quickly between efforts and wanted to treat the equipment like a barbell—badly. Jones summed up the comprehension of their like: *"One advanced bodybuilder asked me as I was trying to explain the machines to him . . . 'Do you have to be a genius to use the machine?' And I told him . . . 'No, but it helps if you are not an idiot.'"*

Barbells CANNOT deliver full-range resistance to working muscles and they're not alone. Multi-exercise pulley stations (and some conventional machines) "redirect" the force of gravity through a series of pulleys. The direction of gravity is ultimately defined by the direction of the cable as it exits the final pulley to connect to a body part. In *all* cases and regardless of direction, the line is straight; and in *all* cases joint movement remains rotational. The result is the same deficient delivery to the working muscles—this time from a different direction.

The popularity of such machines is driven by the current craze for something "functional" and the number and variety of available exercises—none of which provide the requirements of full-range exercise, a fact that was evident more than forty years ago. *"How many people you can stuff in a phone booth is irrelevant,"* said Jones about the Universal® multi-station frenzy of his day. *"Once you set the record, try and use the phone."* There was, and still is, NO regard to function—despite the fancy name.

> **You can't negotiate a curve in the road by driving in a straight line.**

In my humble opinion:

- Barbells are better than most conventional (multi-station) machines.
- The use of resistance beyond free-weights and quality exercise machines—bands, balls, bodyweight—is a step or three backwards especially when better tools are available. If you had a Bentley® and a bicycle in your garage, would you *always* ride the bike?
- Trainees make choices based on ease and current trends—at the moment, skill-based activities.

When Jones revealed his take on the evolution of resistance, "the four steps," he understood that his audience was limited: *". . . Since the average person is too lazy to even do calisthenics, and most people are too lazy to do gymnastics, and even almost all weight-trainees are too lazy to use a barbell in an actually 'hard' fashion, I do not expect very many people to quickly accept and practice a form of training that makes them all seem like child's play by comparison."* [1]

Without harping on the subject, child's play is the precise direction the field of exercise has taken.

My humble opinion faces an uphill climb. Despite the claimed advantages of quality machines, research shows no difference in strength results between the use of free-weights and machines. A recent summary from a reputable British group concluded: *"All resistance types (e.g. free-weights, resistance machines, bodyweight, etc.) show potential for increases in strength, with no significant difference between them, although resistance machines appear to pose a lower risk of injury."* [2]

The summary also singled out a claim of the American College of Sports Medicine that . . . *"free-weights are better than machines for enhancing strength,"* due to reported neural activation. The British reply was swift: *"This recommendation by the ACSM is indicative of a bias toward free-weight resistance forms, which is not justified by the scientific evidence."*

The ACSM also believes that free-weights are superior to machines for sports-based training due to the freedom of movement to work through different planes, including those that mimic sports movements themselves.

That claim CANNOT and WILL NEVER BE substantiated, as you will later discover.

The ACSM is an influential entity that certifies trainers worldwide. Their philosophical stance may be the driving force behind the current trend to diminish the importance and use of individual exercise stations in fitness centers—a pity and pathetic at that.

As mentioned, the heart remains ignorant of the source of the signals it receives. So too, muscle fibers don't recognize the difference between types of resistance. They contract or they don't. If I handed a blindfolded trainee a bale of hay every day and made it weigh a little more each time, his muscles would respond by growing in size and strength—which takes me back to the research summary.

I find it hard to accept as true that research does *not* support the superiority of cam-driven machines. I was brought up to believe otherwise, have "experienced" the difference and am convinced of the accuracy of the results produced in the early days of Nautilus:

- The training that led to the spectacular victory of Casey Viator in the 1971 AAU "Mr. America" competition (brief, hard and infrequent workouts with both free-weights and machines).
- The 1974 "Colorado Experiment" where Viator again demonstrated his extraordinary genetic potential through the use of "machines only."
- The 1975 "Project Total Conditioning" experiment that produced results so superior to the traditional that the West Point staff could not believe them (again, with cam-driven machines).

The results of Viator's victory had to be witnessed to be believed. I was not there but saw photos. The results of the other two experiments were measured by competent, independent groups and left little doubt: Nautilus machines worked muscles harder, but there may have been a second factor at play. Ellington Darden witnessed the final "incredible" workout Viator performed two days prior to the 1971 contest and commented, *"It was hard to distinguish what percentage of the results was produced by the workout, and what percentage was produced by the prodding of Arthur Jones."*

Jones had a way of motivating subjects that was second to none. He could extract every morsel of energy you had—could get your grandmother to momentary failure. Whatever it took he did, and most knew it was coming. He made subjects work harder than they had ever before—a dose of motivation that was probably absent in the cited research studies. Another significant factor: The measurement of strength in research is rarely full-range.

Nonetheless, choice of resistance boils down to preference: But machines remain superior from the perspectives of efficiency and safety. As the Brits concluded, *"How one trains is much more important than the equipment used."* [2]

To add, Nautilus Sports/Medical Industries sold barbells throughout their history.

REFERENCES

[1] Jones, A., *Nautilus Training Principles Bulletin No. 2*, 18: 49, 1971.

[2] Fisher, J., Steele, J., Bruce-Low, S., Smith, D., "Evidence-Based Resistance Training Recommendations," *Medicina Sportiva*, Med Sport 15 (3): 147-162, 2011.

CHAPTER 10

Practical Application

Basic Training-Design

L et's put the puzzle together. First, select four to six lower-body exercises and six to eight upper-body exercises for a total of twelve exercises. If you have no idea what to choose or how to choose, read on. If you have a basic idea, be specific: Your focus is *large* muscle groups and whole-body workouts. Next, select the tool that best meets the needs of the muscle groups or exercises selected according to two criteria: quality of resistance and range of motion over which the resistance is effective. Consider ease of entry, ease of use and your physical status (general health, physical condition, injuries, etc.). *The lower- and upper-body division that follows is purely journalistic.*

Lower Body

Every workout should include exercise for the large muscles of the lower body, the muscles that get you from A to B: those that extend the hip (called "glutes"), the front thigh ("quadriceps"), the rear thigh ("hamstrings") and lower leg ("calves"). The small muscles that abduct, adduct and flex the hip should be considered of minor significance unless they play a crucial role in an activity of interest.

The best (and often only) choices for "**glute**" exercise in gyms are (in no particular order): a butt blaster (one-legged hip extension from an "all-fours" position), leg press, squats (in various forms) and lunges. Butt blasters are scarce and not user-friendly with an aging clientele. Leg press machines have universal appeal and are generally safe—with one caution: They compress the spine when loaded and may lead to back issues. Squats are the most productive exercise for the lower body but feature the same element of risk—spinal compression. The alternative to mounting a heavy barbell on your shoulders—holding dumbbells at your sides—is better for the low back but barely productive. The large muscles that perform squats can handle heavy loads, far more than you can hold in your hands. The same with lunges: As heavy as you can safely handle, both remain as much a cardiovascular trial as a muscle challenge.

Regardless of choice—squats, leg presses and lunges suffer the same shortcoming: There is little to no resistance available when the muscles reach a theoretical position of contraction. If you "lock" your legs at the end of the lift, the muscles might as well take lunch. The weight is transferred to the bones in no productive way. The rapid change of leverage inherent in the movement demands attention to form. ONLY a slow speed during execution will kill the momentum common to all three and allow trainees to "feel" the point at which the resistance tails off (a point about 3-6 inches shy of full extension). Push slowly to that point and change direction immediately without pause to keep tension on the muscles.

Arthur Jones understood the rapid and dramatic change of resistance required to satisfy the muscles during a leg press or squat and stated that its proper application would require a cam *"14-feet high and shaped like a banana."* The upright prototype squat machine he used in "Project Total Conditioning" required the removal of ceiling panels to avoid head injuries. He eventually designed a "reverse" cam that moved in the opposite direction during exercise—the smaller the cam, the more rapid the change of resistance—and applied it to his Duo-Squat machine. The "feel" wasn't kind or popular. Brutal never is.

Something can be salvaged from the low productivity of dumbbell squats and lunges to the pending danger of heavy squats or presses—and it is best accomplished by the wise use of a leg press. The heavy loads required to stimulate the large muscles of the lower body can be reduced without diminishing the productivity of the exercise, as follows:

1. Pre-exhaust muscles before the leg press. Tired muscles can't lift maximum weights. More specifically, perform a leg extension, leg curl or hip extension exercise IMMEDIATELY BEFORE a leg press—and move QUICKLY from one to the other to necessitate a reduction in the resistance.
2. Perform the leg press one leg at a time with slightly more than half of the two-leg weight. This idea can be effectively combined with the next suggestion. For safety, assure that the hip of your working leg aligns with your foot placement on the leg-press platform.
3. Perform the leg press slowly—lift in ten seconds, lower in five—with one leg or two. Select a reduced resistance by trial and error. The suggested speed is only a springboard—you can go as slowly as you'd like provided you don't "linger" near extension.

The **front thigh** muscle is misunderstood: Exercise for the quadriceps has, in many cases, been deflected to compound movements such as those described above, despite the FACT that the best way to strengthen the front thigh to its potential is through the use of a Leg Extension machine. Figure 1 (below) clarifies the supposed and often declared danger(s) associated with the use of the tool.

To start, the knee is the most mechanically inefficient joint system in the body. To lift 100 pounds, the front thigh must pull with a force of 1,200 pounds. The effective pull (output) is reduced by 200 pounds due to internal muscle friction and by another 80% due to its point of attachment with the lower leg (B), where the direction of pull is poor. The reduced output—by now, 200 pounds—is then cut in half because the effective point of attachment (C) is twice as far below the knee's rotational axis.

That's the good news.

Figure 1:

THE MECHANICAL INEFFICIENCY OF THE KNEE

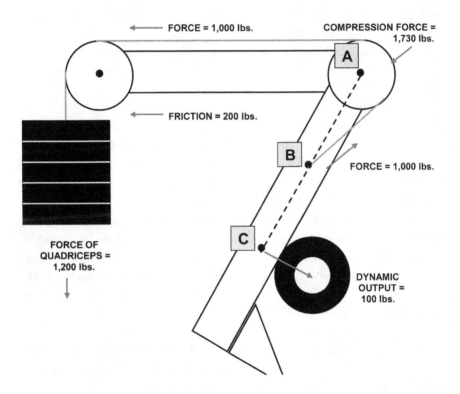

FORCE = 1,000 lbs.

COMPRESSION FORCE = 1,730 lbs.

A

FRICTION = 200 lbs.

B

FORCE = 1,000 lbs.

FORCE OF QUADRICEPS = 1,200 lbs.

C

DYNAMIC OUTPUT = 100 lbs.

At the start of a leg-extension movement (approximately 120°, as illustrated), the knee is exposed to a compression force that is 73% higher than the pulling force of the muscles. When legs are bent at 90°, the compression force is 40% higher; and at 66° short of full extension, only 9%. *"When fully extended, straight,"* according to Jones' grade-school math and physics, *"the magnification of force is zero."*

In plain English leg extensions are more dangerous at the bottom (the start of the movement) than at the top. The top position is undeniably safe: The muscles are NOT exposed to more force than they can produce. The disagreement lies in "how it feels" from a muscle perspective. Eight repetitions in with a tough weight can make a grown man cry and failure will make him cry ON THE FLOOR. As Jones put it, *"If you can walk after performing one set of leg extensions, you didn't do it right."*

Productive it is—dangerous it is not (certainly not as perceived). I credit my lack of knee problems to the performance of heavy leg extensions for forty years and believe that most trainees can perform them without issues. I am also aware that certain knee conditions are contraindicated. Check with a doctor or therapist before you start, but do them if you can during most workouts. There's more to gain than lose.

The rear thigh or "**hamstrings**" cannot be exercised in a meaningful way without the use of either a prone or seated leg-curl machine. The less common prone version was phased out by complaints of low-back problems that surfaced when the muscles reached a contracted position causing the back to arch. At the time Nautilus advocated arching the back to increase range of motion, and it did. But complaints continued. Manufacturers shaped the machine's cushion to prevent or support the arch but eventually moved to the seated version. One day I asked Dr. Fulton (orthopedic representative for Nautilus) if the new edition decreased or eliminated low-back issues. *"No difference,"* he claimed. There was also no difference in results or downsides.

Prone leg-curl units struggle to deliver a challenging resistance in the final angles of contraction because the direction of the movement arm—by then—is horizontal. Seated versions present issues with entry and comfort. Nonetheless, use whatever is available. The importance of rear-thigh muscles to performance, injury prevention and knee stability is undeniable.

> **If you can walk after performing one set of leg extensions, you didn't do it right.**

Calf muscles are often ignored because their importance is rarely linked to function. Calves combine with front- and rear-thigh muscles to stabilize the knee.

Despite that, Arthur Jones refused to build a calf machine. The simple action of raising the heels to a tip-toe position produced a strength curve that was "too-close-to-perfect" to justify the addition of a cam. Calf machines exist but the job can be done without them: All you need is a raised surface (a step or block of wood) and a dumbbell. Start with two legs (no weight) and gradually progress to one while holding a dumbbell. Calves are strong in a standing position and can lift as much weight as you can hold. If your facility has calf machines, avoid those with shoulder pads that compress the spine. And caution: Calf exercise initially produces more muscle soreness than other exercises. Ease your way in. One set. Twice a week.

To summarize, the leg section of a whole-body workout should list as follows:

- Leg Extension
- Leg Press
- Leg Curl
- Calf Raise

Minor lower-body muscle groups (hip abduction, hip adduction and hip flexion) can be added if you chose to perform more than four.

Do NOT add a balance factor to basic lower-body exercises. Your purpose is to stimulate growth, not win a blue ribbon.

Upper Body

Training the upper body affords six to eight exercise choices—more muscles to choose from. At the forefront are chest, shoulders and upper back. Common exercises for the three are listed below:

	Direct Exercises	**Indirect (Multi-Joint) Exercises**
CHEST	Chest Fly (dumbbells)	Chest Press
	Pec-Dec (machine)	Dip
UPPER BACK	Pullover (machine)	Pull-down, Chin-Up
		Rowing
SHOULDERS	Lateral and Front Raise	Shoulder Press
	Rear Deltoid (reverse fly)	

The direct exercises (above) involve rotation around one axis, the shoulder joint. The indirect exercises involve rotation around more than one axis—shoulder and elbow joints—which activates the smaller muscles of the upper arm. Indirect chest and shoulder movements involve pushing with triceps; upper-back movements, pulling with biceps.

Once you complete your lower-body exercises, begin working the upper-body with either shoulder or chest exercises, followed by upper-back and then, by whatever remains. That is:

- SHOULDER / Upper-Back / CHEST *or*
- CHEST / Upper-Back / SHOULDER.

Why?—to avoid too many or consecutive exercises that involve the use of triceps.

Select one or two exercises from each upper-body muscle group. If you select two, perform the direct exercise first, then the indirect. The direct exercise exhausts the major muscle; the indirect further works the same muscle with the help of the arms. Sample torso sequences follow:

1. Lateral raise, shoulder press / pullover, pull-down / chest fly, chest press.
2. Chest fly, dip / chin-up / front raise.
3. Lateral raise / pull-down / chest press / rowing.

Several notes:

- Shoulder presses compress the spine. When possible, exhaust the shoulders prior to performing presses to reduce the resistance and risk.
- Pullover machines provide the ONLY direct exercise for the upper back but are rare to gyms. Ask the staff for identification and instruction.
- Perform pull-downs and chin-ups with a palms-up or parallel grip (palms facing each other) so the muscles likely to fatigue first (biceps) can provide the upper-back muscles a few more reps. A palms-down grip, the weakest, should be used sparingly. Grip width is equally significant: Wide reduces the range of motion and should be avoided, as should pulls behind the neck.
- Chest flys and chest presses are tough on shoulders. Presses, in particular, jam the upper-arm into the joint. Ease into heavier weights, restrict the distance you lower the resistance and ALWAYS move slowly toward a stretch position.
- Select enough indirect upper-body exercises to include biceps and triceps at least once.
- Do NOT add a balance factor to basic upper-body exercises.

Upon completion of the upper-body, proceed to arms. If your final torso exercise involved biceps (as Example #3, above), begin arm training with triceps. If your final torso exercise involved triceps (as Example #1, above), begin with biceps. If the final torso exercise was direct and involved neither biceps nor triceps (as Example #2 above), select either biceps or triceps to start, as follows:

1. Lateral raise, shoulder press / pullover, pull-down / chest fly, chest press / biceps / triceps.
2. Chest fly, dip / chin-up / front raise / triceps / biceps (or biceps / triceps).
3. Lateral raise / pull-down / chest press / rowing / triceps / biceps.

Do NOT add a balance factor to basic lower-body or upper-body exercises. Your purpose is to stimulate growth, not win a blue ribbon.

At this point, count the number of exercises and keep the limit to twelve. Why not more—another exercise, another set? Probably nothing on occasion, but sticking to twelve (or less) has advantages. The first is physiological. Twelve, properly performed, is enough to stimulate growth (remember the trail of bodies on the floor in Lake Helen, Florida?) and about all you can stand. The second is psychological. Presented with limited opportunity, you tend to "up your game."

The mindset of performing a prolonged versus brief amount of exercise during a workout is unique. An unlimited amount generates a "go-through-the-motions" approach; whereas, a limited number of exercises is more likely to produce an aggressive approach and, ultimately, the level of intensity necessary to stimulate change. Jones set the limit at twelve.

The remaining exercises (of twelve) can be performed by small muscles of choice—neck, forearms, low back, abdominals, obliques—at the end of the workout.

The basic, whole-body workouts that follow are samples (the combinations are endless):

A. Leg Extension, Leg Curl, Leg Press, Calf Raise, Hip Abduction, Lateral Raise, Shoulder Press, Pullover, Chin-ups, Chest Fly, Chest Press, Biceps Curls.
B. Leg Curl, Leg Extension, Squats, Calf Raise, Chest Press, Pull-downs, Shoulder Press, Rowing, Dips, Biceps Curls, Triceps Extensions, Wrist Curls.
C. Leg Extension, Leg Press, Leg Curl, Squats, Hip Adduction, Calf Raise, Chin-ups, Chest press, Lateral Raise, Triceps Extensions, Biceps Curls, Abdomen Curls.

Arthur Jones believed that outstanding results could be achieved by a handful of basic free-weight exercises continued to a point of momentary fatigue. He outlined a sample program in his 1971 publication, *Nautilus Training Principles Bulletin No. 2*. At the time, he advocated performing two sets of some exercises, as follows:

- Full squats (1 set of 20 repetitions)
- One-leg Calf Raises (1 set of 20 repetitions)
- Standing (shoulder) Press (1 set of 10 repetitions)
- Palms-up Chin-ups (1 set of 10 repetitions)
- Standing (shoulder) Press (a second set of 10 repetitions)
- Palms-up Chin-ups (a second set of 10 repetitions)
- Parallel Bar Dips (1 set of 10 repetitions)
- Standing Biceps Curls (1 set of 10 repetitions)
- Parallel Bar Dips (a second set of 10 repetitions)
- Standing Biceps Curls (a second set of 10 repetitions)
- Deadlifts (1 set of 15 repetitions)

The suggested routine contained seven different exercises, a total of eleven sets and represented much less exercise than what was traditionally performed by bodybuilders. *"There will be a natural temptation to do 'more'—to add sets, or new exercises;"* he said, *"but fastest growth will result if the program is performed exactly as outlined."* [1]

He also explained what to expect. *"Beginning trainees gain faster than advanced trainees in almost all cases for a very simple reason—simply because their strength levels are such that they don't entirely use up their recovery ability in each workout. Later, when they get stronger, they DO use up all of their recovery ability—and growth stops."* [2]

Advanced training requires less exercise.

There will be a natural temptation to do 'more'—to add sets, or new exercises; but fastest growth will result if the program is performed exactly as outlined.

Advanced Training

Without defining "advanced," a reduction in training frequency is warranted when workouts begin to deplete your recovery ability and progress stalls (determined by workout records) You might "feel" good but numbers don't lie. When you compare workouts, compare identical sequences, perhaps a favorite you perform every other week or month. In the beginning it normally takes a few weeks to acquire good form, a few months to reach levels of intensity required to stimulate growth and several more to reach a plateau. After approximately 4-6 months, you may require a reduction in training.

Progress occurs in spurts and there are a two ways to deal with plateaus: Make exercise harder and/or allow the body more time to recover.

In his 2004 book, *The New High Intensity Training*, Ellington Darden dedicated a chapter to techniques that expose muscles to greater levels of intensity:

- Cheating repetitions
- Forced repetitions
- Breakdown sets
- 1 ¼ repetitions
- Stage repetitions
- Pre-exhaustion sets
- Negative repetitions
- Super-slow repetitions
- Extremely slow repetitions

It's not my intent to elaborate here: All are effective when properly applied and several require no outside assistance. The prerequisites to make exercise harder relate to sequence, muscle-fiber recruitment and pace.

Exercise Sequence

Simple adjustments to sequence can make a significant difference in workout intensity. One such adjustment can lead to what are called "pre-exhaustion" routines as exemplified by the upper-body sequence of Basic Routine A (above). The goal of pre-exhaustion is to force a fatigued muscle to immediately perform a second exercise with "fresh" help. For example, the pullover/chin-up combination of Routine A forces tired upper-back muscles (from the Pullover) to greater fatigue with help from fresh biceps (chin-ups are considered a back *and* biceps exercise). The net effect creates a greater inroad.

For best results with pre-exhaustion combinations, restrict time between exercises to less than three seconds. To facilitate the time restraint, Jones constructed several "double" machines that allowed two exercises from one seat: The Nautilus Compound Leg (leg extension/leg press), Double Shoulder (lateral raise/shoulder press), Double Chest (chest fly/chest press), Pullover/Torso Arm (pullover/pull-down) and Behind Neck/Torso Arm (behind-neck pullover/behind-neck pull-down). The combinations took such a toll that recommended use was limited to no more than two per routine. Today's manufacturers don't make double machines which limits pre-exhaustion to moving quickly from a single station to another single station. Both stations must be "ready-to-go" to pull it off. Less than three seconds is FAST.

Pre-exhaustion combinations include:

- LEGS—Leg Extension IMMEDIATELY followed by Leg Press or Squat (barbell).
- SHOULDERS—Lateral Raise IMMEDIATELY followed by Shoulder Press.
- UPPER BACK—Pullover (machine) IMMEDIATELY followed by Pull-down to front or Chin-ups (palm up).
- CHEST—Chest Fly IMMEDIATELY followed by Chest Press (free-weights or machine).
- BICEPS—Biceps Curls IMMEDIATELY followed by Negative Chin-ups.
- TRICEPS—Triceps Extensions IMMEDIATELY followed by Negative Dips.

No more than two combinations should be included in a routine of ten total exercises—and no more than twice a week.

Non-stop **triple combinations** are also possible, as follows:

- LEGS—Leg Press/ Leg Extension/ Squat (a favorite of Arthur's).
- SHOULDERS—Lateral Raise/ Upright Row/ Shoulder Press.
- UPPER BACK—Pull-down/ Pullover (machine)/ Bent-over or Seated Row; Pull-down/ Pullover (machine)/ Negative Chin-ups.
- CHEST—Chest Press/ Chest Fly/ Negative Dips.
- BICEPS—Chin-ups/ Biceps curls (barbell)/ Negative Chin-ups.
- TRICEPS—Chest Press/ Triceps Extensions/ Negative Dips.

The middle and final exercises of each triple combination require a reduction of as much as 40-50% of the resistance normally used, but instructions for its effective use are the same: No more than two triple combinations in a routine of ten exercises—and no more than twice a week.

Another effective and easy-to-design sequence is called "Push/Pull"—you push during one exercise and pull on the next, alternating through a choice of exercises that stimulates major muscle groups. Sample Basic Workout B (above) has elements of Push/Pull and resembles the routine I used with first-time bodybuilders in Venezuela:

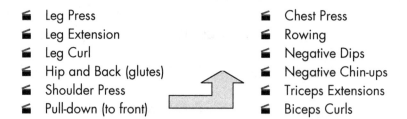

- Leg Press
- Leg Extension
- Leg Curl
- Hip and Back (glutes)
- Shoulder Press
- Pull-down (to front)

- Chest Press
- Rowing
- Negative Dips
- Negative Chin-ups
- Triceps Extensions
- Biceps Curls

Few made it.

Muscle-Fiber Recruitment

Strength gain is related to the number of muscle fibers involved in an exercise—the more the merrier. But intensity of effort, the major determining factor, is only part of the story. The ONLY position that allows maximum recruitment of fibers is that of full contraction. The combination of high intensity and a full-contracted position can be achieved by the performance of 1¼-repetitions on exercise machines that provide adequate resistance in the contracted position.

Let's use Leg Extension as an example. Set the machine as normal—same settings and weight. Lift the weight to the top position and PAUSE momentarily. Slowly lower the weight about one quarter of the way down. From there, reverse direction and slowly lift the weight again to the top. PAUSE. Lower the weight to the original starting position: One full lift, followed by a one-quarter lift; and repeat until movement is no longer possible.

The 1¼-technique reduces the possible number of repetitions. Its effectiveness lies in the fact that, on the road to fatigue, the muscle spends more time near or in a position of full contraction. This triggers the recruitment of more muscle fibers during the effort.

The application of this technique is limited to exercises that provide resistance in a contracted position. With few exceptions free-weight exercises do not. Machine exercises that push away from the body's center (squats, presses and dips) are not good candidates: A pause in contraction during such exercises represents a rest. You can rest at home.

Perform a workout that includes as many 1¼-repetition exercises as possible (in a ten-exercise routine) or work the technique into a normal session. In either case, keep accurate records to gauge progress.

Pace

A lot has been made of a training system called Super-Slow,® developed by former Nautilus employee, Ken Hutchins. Motivated by the momentum he witnessed during exercise, Hutchins believed that too little emphasis was placed on execution. His solution: time each repetition—ten seconds to lift, ten seconds to lower. To keep total time within productive parameters, Super-Slow favors a repetition range of four to six.

A slower pace of movement during exercise makes resistance "feel" heavier which sends a signal to recruit help. To add, the muscle is forced to work through the range of motion *without* momentum. Super-Slow facilities around the country package their product to a limited but loyal audience: Limited, because it follows the philosophical approach of hard, brief and infrequent; loyal, because it works. Despite that, some don't like the rigidity of the system, the sterile environment offered by some facilities and the large clock "in your face" at every station.

Super-Slow training is best performed with machines—but not all machines are appropriate. Friction reduces the effectiveness of slow movement and the average machine creates too much friction as it moves. Friction makes the lifting phase feel heavier and the lowering phase feel lighter, reducing tension on the muscle. To combat the problem, Hutchins modified already-low-friction machines to satisfy the needs of his system.

Typical gym machines work if they are new. If not, MedX machines, new or old, are your best choice: Their friction is the lowest in the market. The twenty MedX tools we have in Florida are smoother—at twelve-years old—than many of today's new tools.

A slow cadence can be applied to an entire workout or to a few exercises within a workout. If it is implemented in a complete full-body session, perform no more than eight exercises and limit frequency to once a week. If several exercises per workout are incorporated, perform no more than four super-slow movements in a single workout and train no more than twice per week.

It doesn't sound like much, but Super-Slow will get your attention.

Beyond Failure

The "bench press" is the most popular yet worst-performed exercise in gyms: Big guys with arched backs bouncing heavy barbells off their chest—a grunt on the lift, locked elbows, a few forced exhalations, a quick drop of the weight and a rebound off the chest. When the bar reaches the bottom with speed, shoulders are exposed to a force several times the weight of the bar—just part of the show.

Danger aside, trainees are missing the boat. Arthur Jones did not invent negative work (lowering weight as a form of exercise) but brought it to the forefront in the early 1970's. Lowering weight is more important than lifting. The controlled lowering of resistance sets up a stretch when the muscle reaches an extended position, can trigger a pre-stretch (which activates more muscle fibers) in the same extended position, can be used to strengthen an injured or atrophied muscle and can further stimulate a muscle that has reached momentary failure. Despite all the "good," it remains ignored.

And for good reason: It "feels" harder to lift than lower a weight and trainees wrongly equate that to the production of results.

The "feel" is real. Muscles are 40% stronger lowering than lifting under "fresh" conditions—the difference due to internal muscle friction created by fibers sliding across one another during movement. Jones demonstrated the phenomenon with an isokinetic leg-extension machine that measured front-thigh strength—both lifting and lowering—during every repetition. On one test, the subject's pre-exercise ratio of lifting to lowering strength was 1: 1.4. He was 40% stronger lowering than lifting when his muscle was "fresh." The final repetition (his twenty-fifth) displayed a ratio of 1: 57. The subject was 5,700% stronger lowering than lifting when his front thigh was totally fatigued. From the thirteenth repetition on, his lifting strength plummeted while his lowering strength increased—a demonstration of increased internal muscle friction.

The point is simple: When a muscle can no longer lift, it can still lower. And if it lowers a resistance to failure, it creates an inroad greater than lifting a resistance to failure.

To make good use of the fact, Jones came up with three techniques that led to failure during negative work: Negative Emphasis, Negative Accentuated and Negative Only.

Negative Emphasis

Negative-emphasis exercise involves lifting a weight in a normal fashion and having a buddy or trainer push against the movement arm or weight as it lowers: Lift the weight and resist the added push as it lowers. This increases the inroad and the total work performed per set. The task requires external assistance which introduces variables—a search for help and a reliable, smooth push. From the helper's perspective, it's difficult to judge how hard to push. The only indicators are "feel" and the speed of the movement arm. In either case, the force applied cannot be measured in an accurate way from session to session which makes long-term progress next to impossible. There is also a risk with the manual application of resistance. A slight hesitation on the part of the trainer or trainee could result in a sudden acceleration or deceleration—the definition of injury.

With negative-emphasis exercise, reduce the standard weight by 30% and select a machine with a fused movement arm (one that requires the use of both limbs together). Lift normally, lower in eight to ten seconds and continue until the act of lowering cannot be controlled. Because of the inherent danger and the inability to measure progress, use this technique sporadically with any exercise or use it to surpass plateaus on specific exercises.

Negative Accentuated

Negative-accentuated exercise involves lifting a resistance with two limbs and lowering with one. Select a machine with a fused movement arm and reduce the weight by 40%. Lift the weight slowly to a contracted position and carefully remove one limb. Slowly lower the weight in eight to ten seconds. Lift with both limbs again and lower with the opposite limb. Continue alternating limbs until lifting becomes impossible or lowering lacks control. The goal is to lift for twelve repetitions and lower for six with each limb. When the weight transfers to one limb for the descent, it represents 120% of what you would normally lower.

This style of training requires no help and allows measurable progress. The only negative is obvious: While one limb works the other rests and that, combined with the accumulation of internal muscle friction may lead to the frustration of slow failure. During my initial exposure to negative-accentuated exercise, I kept going and going and thought that the weight was too light, or that my form was bad. But bad form is nearly impossible when lowering weight—a good thing. I was equally surprised by how sore I became days after the effort. For physiological reasons that remain unknown, negative work—performed in any style—produces more muscle soreness than traditional positive/negative training.

Negative Only

Negative-only exercise is the hardest and most productive form of training. It requires the use of weights 40% heavier than normal and a cast of assistants to lift it—you lower. Eventually the resistance required for strong trainees exceeds the capacity of the assistants. Jones performed negative-only exercise with bodybuilders and football players in the 1970's with great success, but had to abandon several exercises due to the risk of transferring heavy weights safely to the trainee.

To solve the problem he built machines that used the strongest muscles of the body (hips and legs) to lift a heavy weight that was then lowered by upper-body muscles (chest, shoulders, arms). He marketed only a few of his tools due to friction and impracticality—but one became a "hit." The Nautilus Multi-Exercise machine offered, among other exercises, the possibility of negative-only chin-ups and dips.

From day one, Jones recognized the value and difficulty of both exercises. He built three steps in front of an adjustable chin/dip bar that allowed trainees to ascend to a contracted position using legs and then lower using arms. The machine featured a waist-belt that clipped to its weight-stack. It looked easy but was not. Ten negative chin-ups to failure left everyone looking as if they had just completed a 100-meter Olympic final.

Both exercises can be performed by using a bench or set of aerobic steps under a chin-up or dip bar. Step to the top position, remove your legs, lower slowly in eight to ten seconds and quickly return to the top. Do not jump to the starting position, especially as fatigue sets in. Continue to lower until lowering occurs in less than three seconds or you can't safely control the descent. You may need a spotter.

The use of a chin/dip assist station found in gyms is inappropriate for negative-only work. The platforms are generally too low to allow you to safely reach an upper starting position.

Besides that, Arthur Jones had a low opinion of anything that assisted the lifting phase of exercise. Long after the introduction of the Multi-Exercise machine, Dr. Fulton, who had one, decided to purchase a Gravitron®

(a chin/dip assist station) for his showcase rehabilitation center. The jaw-dropping facility served as host to Jones' potential medical clients and was located across from the Daytona International Speedway on a site formerly occupied by a high-end bar. As soon as the new hydraulic monster was installed, the phone rang. Arthur was on his way with guests.

Fulton decided to usher the entourage through an auxiliary entrance far removed from the Gravitron—prudent, but without effect. The moment he entered, Jones was drawn to the hard-to-miss tower like a magnet and approached with a floor-to-ceiling scan. "Mike," he said, "what the hell is this?" Fulton described its function in as few words as possible but Arthur was equally curt. He turned and walked away, mumbling as he went, "Piece of Sh—, Piece of Sh—."

A greater inroad could be made HIS WAY.

Negative work is difficult to recover from and must be used infrequently. Regardless of style, one set of negative exercise per body part per week is the general recommendation. More is *not* better—and there's proof.

When Jones introduced the potential of negative work to the bodybuilding community, many professionals began to perform *every* set of *every* exercise at *every* workout in a negative style and then bashed it publically. It "didn't work," which led Arthur to comment, "*If race horses were trained as much as most bodybuilders train, you could safely bet your money on an out-of-condition turtle— it would be unlikely that a horse trained in such a fashion could even make it around the track, and certainly not rapidly.*"

Negative work deserves respect.

For physiological reasons that remain unknown, negative work, performed in any style, produces more muscle soreness than traditional positive/negative training.

Summary

The above guidelines represent a start. How you perform exercise is more important than how you put things together. It was not my intent to be specific: There are plenty of opinions and specifics out there.

The debate between high-intensity and high-volume training rages on with each camp taking a stand and digging in. My preference continues to be the former. If the prime goal is the same—to maximize physical potential—and the end result the same (as it generally is), I prefer its efficiency, logic and physiologic sense.

And no small point—it evolved from the greatest mind in the field of exercise.

REFERENCES

[1] Jones, A., *Nautilus Training Principles Bulletin No. 2*, 34: 106, 1971.

[2] Jones, A., *Nautilus Training Principles Bulletin No. 2*, 35: 109, 1971.

PART II

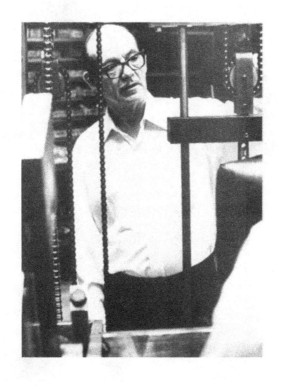

The Courtesy Flush

CHAPTER 11

....

Motor Learning

In the late 1960's my Physical Education degree included study of a subject that has long been ignored in the field of exercise—Motor Learning—in essence, how we learn movement skills. A basic understanding of its concepts is crucial to a discussion of current trends in exercise. To start, let's define two commonly misunderstood terms: *abilities* and *skills*.

A *skill* is a specific movement learned in life (climbing stairs, ice skating, throwing a baseball, combing your hair, sinking a three-foot putt, etc.). Some skills require no conscious thought (*are part of a general motor program*) while others require regular and specific practice. With practice, some people acquire a high level of proficiency (*make it look easy*), while others, with all the practice in the world, verify what Arthur Jones believed: *"You can't train a donkey for the Kentucky Derby."*

The elements and characteristics of a skill are unique and specific unto themselves—a concept known as "specificity." No two skills are alike.

Every skill is supported by a base of stable traits called *abilities* that are genetically determined early in the maturation process and *not* subject to change through practice. Abilities are pre-structured commands that act as an "executive" motor program within the spinal cord. Their activation results in fundamental actions that take place automatically without direct or conscious control. Linked together, they determine how well motor tasks are performed from a general perspective but do not provide specific skill patterns. To reach one's performance potential requires maximizing specific skills which are supported by abilities that have reached their peak.

In broad physical terms, abilities encompass the following capacities: *Strength, power and speed* (all genetically limited but enhanced by greater muscle mass and skill proficiency), *cardiovascular endurance and flexibility* (genetically limited but increased through training specifics) and *agility, coordination and balance* (genetically determined but *not* subject to change). The contribution of each of the general abilities (*strength, power, speed, endurance, flexibility, agility, coordination and balance*) varies from one task to another. A particular skill, for example, may require an emphasis on balance with a minimal focus on speed or endurance. Another may require the opposite.

This supports two notions: That proficiency in one activity does not ensure proficiency in another, and that practice of one activity has no influence on the skill proficiency of another since the requirements of the involved abilities (*balance, agility, strength, etc.*) are dissimilar. An individual may lack the proper combination of abilities to be proficient or "as proficient" in a second task, which explains why a set of skills within a task WILL NOT, and CANNOT, transfer to another. The fact that common (*similar*) abilities underlie the performance of different tasks makes people think there is a crossover of skills. But skills and abilities are different and no such crossover exists.

How We Learn

As we learn and refine a motor skill, numerous stages of information processing take place: FIRST, the identification of the stimulus (input) via sensory perception; SECOND, the selection of an appropriate response; THIRD, the programming/organization of the motor system to produce the desired movement and complete the task; and FOURTH, the output, which may or may not achieve the intended goal.

INPUT

Most of the input during the learning process (and memory retrieval) is based on sensory perception—what can be seen, heard, tasted, smelled and touched. The feedback from these sensors delivers a unique set of instructions to the brain to control movement according to the specific goals of the task. The major sensors involved include:

- Muscle spindles—tiny sensors located between, and connected in-parallel-to, muscle fibers. They determine the position and velocity of body parts and are sensitive to muscle length (send a signal to "contract" when muscle reaches its stretch limit or approaches that limit with too much speed).
- Golgi tendon organs—minute receptors located at the muscle/tendon junction that provide information about tension in the muscle and reduce it, when needed, to prevent injury.
- Joint receptors—located within joint capsules to indicate position (their role in movement is unknown).
- Cutaneous receptors—located in the skin to process information about touch and pressure.

All sensors work together to indicate the position of the body, establish movement patterns and maintain equilibrium (that is, sustain a center of gravity within a support base). The process is ongoing—the system compares feedback it receives during movement to feedback it expects to receive and attempts to correct discrepancies on the go. Compensation is based on length-tension relationships of body parts to create appropriate stabilization, movement and the most efficient completion of the task.

Sensors do not produce movement but play an important role in accuracy when movement is slow. Fast movements happen so quickly that proper form must be established before, and mistakes corrected after, the event.

RESPONSE

The body sorts through the incoming information to determine an appropriate response and produce a desired action—a process that improves with practice. Initially the learning process is rife with problem-solving (physical

---

The elements and characteristics of a skill are unique and specific unto themselves—a concept known as "specificity." No two skills are alike.

---

and mental), inconsistent input and outcome, inefficient movement, errors, indecision, muscle tension, and poor timing and execution. As skills improve the individual becomes more relaxed, certain and decisive; and movement more efficient, fluid, accurate and automatic. The final result depends on motivation, individual ability and prior experiences.

PROGRAMMING

During the learning process the mind integrates the available sensory information with the motor components it intends to use and creates a "blueprint" that makes each activity specific. The blueprint is used only if the execution of the intended action is the SAME as the blueprint suggests. If the action varies (and the blueprint is altered), the exact "integration" requirements of one movement are NOT the same as another. As a result, the new (different) incoming information must be processed and compared to what is known. New skills require learning and therefore have no direct or positive bearing on unlike skills, regardless of how they appear to be similar.

OUTPUT

The result of a specific input, response and program blueprint is a specific output. Each task or skill is as unique as its reflex feedback and motor programming. Consequently, the nature of one task/set of skills is non-specific to another and any transfer of skill (to enhance a seemingly similar but different set of skills) is impossible—and the attempt, as Arthur Jones would say, *"Useless for its intended purpose."*

Specificity

In the mid 1990's I attended a lecture conducted by a triumvirate of exercise heavyweights at the University of Florida: Arthur Jones (Chairman, MedX Corporation), Michael Fulton, M.D. (US Water-Ski Team physician; Orthopedic representative, MedX) and Michael Pollock, Ph.D., (past president, American College of Sports Medicine; Director, Center for Exercise Science,

Colleges of Medicine and Health and Human Performance, University of Florida). During the event, Dr. Pollock referenced a study conducted by my exercise physiology professor at McMaster University. Digby Sale, Ph.D., discovered that the development of muscle hypertrophy was preceded by a neural adaptive phase during the initial stages of strength training. In other words, the nervous system must first master the skill of lifting before it allows the muscle(s) to increase in size and strength. This makes the preliminary progress in strength training due, in large, to enhanced proficiency in skill.

The same applies when muscles are exposed to different types of resistance—they must first master the skill required of the new before they progress in strength. It takes time, for example, to adapt to the feel of free weights if your program is machine-based. Conversely, free-weight trainees struggle with the feel of machines or when first perched on a Swiss ball. Skill mastery of a Nautilus machine will *not* produce instant success on a Cybex machine, although the strength gained through Nautilus training may come in handy.

One fact leaps from motor-learning research—skill is specific to the task. The alteration of ANY element of a movement (*including a change of speed or force imposed upon the involved muscles*) establishes a NEW motor program—a non-specific skill—that the nervous system must identify and process.

Skill practice must be precise, exact—specific. Anything less triggers the selection of new and different pathways, which creates a new and different skill.

Transfer

Skill transfer refers to the attainment (or loss) of proficiency in one task as a result of practice at some other task. According to IART (International Association of Resistance Trainers) President, Brian Johnston, *"It has been demonstrated time and again that positive transfer (in reference to neuromuscular patterning) is either non-existent or quite negligible (negligible among tasks that are almost exactly the same, but slightly different in some regard). The one notable exception . . . is the timing or temporal aspect of* skills. Timing and rhythm of one activity can transfer to similar activities. However, that is insignificant to the application (of skill-based training) within the fitness, athletic, and rehabilitation fields." [1]

The result of a specific stimulus is a specific response. Implementation of a motor pattern that is nearly similar or completely dissimilar does not have a bearing on another skill or demonstration of ability. There is NO correlation, for example, among balance abilities. If a person has difficulty walking due to a balance problem, the problem CANNOT be improved by standing on a wobble board or sprawling over a Swiss ball. Training a general ability called "balance" will NOT improve the balance component of a specific skill. Therefore, exposing yourself (or others) to the danger of training in an unstable environment to improve an abstract skill you may never use borders on insanity—but happens *every* day on the training floor.

FACT ONE: Weak or hampered skills can only be improved *specifically*. You can't improve a golf swing by taking a tennis lesson or something "like" a golf lesson. You take a golf lesson. Why, then, do skill-based trainers insist on the introduction of new skills (often through Swiss-ball exercises) to correct different skills that need improvement?

FACT TWO: Once old skills are in place, it takes a lot of practice to change them. That's because an established skill ingrains itself in the neuromuscular system and is stored for later extraction from a memory bank. A skill that is non-specific to a task makes its own, unique impression in the neuromuscular system and it, too, must be practiced to increase proficiency and establish automatic recall. Therefore, based on the fundamental requirements for retention and extraction, there can be NO transfer of skill . . . but there are false impressions.

The alteration of ANY element of a movement (*including a change of speed or force imposed upon the involved muscles*) establishes a NEW motor program - a non-specific skill - that the nervous system must identify and process.

False positive transfer

Many athletes report an improvement in skill when they modify training to a skill-based system (such as "sport-specific" or "functional" training). This may be due to one or more of the following: increased motivation on the new system, for whatever reason, including the quality of coaching; better recovery from months of intense strength training, since skill-based exercises are less intense than weight-training; different styles of training or nutrition; improved practice of the sport skills; maturation of the individual (the athlete becomes more capable within his or her means); and false research conclusions about the specificity of motor learning and methods of measuring transfer. Two additional points: The reported improvement in condition (and performance) attributed to skill-based training could possibly have been achieved by other methods in less time; and, there are as many successful athletes who do NOT perform skill-based exercises as athletes who do.

Negative Transfer

Negative transfer occurs when learning one skill negatively affects the quality of another—when a skill that appears to be similar is practiced and alters a motor program by creating a hybrid. According to Arthur Jones, the closer the new skill is to the old, the more likely it is to confuse the nervous system. For the most part, negative transfer is small and exists only during initial practice, particularly if the old skills have been well ingrained in memory.

To summarize: With "unlike" activities, there is no positive transfer—and probably no negative transfer; with "like" activities, there is no positive transfer—but a greater probability of negative transfer. Skill-based exercise advocates disagree: They believe that there is positive transfer with "like" AND "unlike" activities—and rarely acknowledge the existence of negative transfer.

Literature and Research

What does Motor-Learning research and literature say about specificity and transfer?

A. "Activities which look similar, but are performed at slightly different speeds, are most likely to be completely dissimilar in their training effects. Every alteration of path of movement or apparatus used is a different neuromuscular pattern of movement development." [2]

B. *"A common misconception is that fundamental abilities (reaction time, movement speed, flexibility, explosive strength and gross-body coordination) can be trained through various drills or other activities. The thinking is that, with some stronger ability, the athlete will see gains in performance for tasks with this underlying ability. For example, athletes are often given quickening exercises, with the hope that these exercises would train some fundamental ability to be quick, allowing quicker responses in their particular sport. Coaches often use various balancing drills to increase general balancing ability, eye movement exercises to improve vision, and many others. Such attempts to train fundamental abilities may sound fine, but usually they simply do not work. Time, and often money, would be better spent practicing the eventual goal skills.*

There are two correct ways to think of these principles. First, there is no general ability to be quick, to balance, or to use vision. Rather, quickness, balance, and vision are each based on many diverse abilities, so there is no single quickness ability, for example, that can be trained. Second, even if there were such general abilities, these are, by definition, genetic and not subject to modification through practice. Therefore, attempts to modify abilities with nonspecific drills are ineffective. A learner may acquire additional skill at the drill (which is a skill itself), but this learning does not transfer to the main skill of interest." [3]

C. "Practice of non-specific coordination or quickening tasks will not produce transfer to specific sport skills. In regards to quickening exercises that involve many rapid skillful movements, transfer of learning is highly specific and occurs only when the practiced movements are identical." [4]

D. *"Minor alterations from an exact action change the characteristics of the systems that produce the altered action. Such changes are potentially harmful to a well-trained athlete."* [5]

E. "When training has occurred through participation in large-muscle total-body activities, such as running, rowing or Olympic lifting, there can be partial but minor transfer of training effects to simpler activities. For example, aerobic improvements derived from running (a complex activity) have been shown to produce improvements in the aerobic work of cycling (a simpler activity where the work occurs in fewer large muscle groups). The amount of transfer is marginal at best. The aerobic benefits that could be derived from 100 hours of endurance running might translate into the equivalent effect of 10 hours of endurance training for cycling. It would seem to be more expedient and economical to just train for 10 hours on a bicycle rather than perform 10 times as much running-training to get an improvement in cycling. As well, cycling produces specific endurance effects plus other associated benefits (which would not result from relying on the transfer of the running-training phenomenon)." [6]

Observations

When I was eight, Dad took me to Fort Erie, Ontario to see a man who became my first sports hero. Eddie Feigner, the pitching sensation of a four-man softball team that barnstormed the country as "The King and his Court," could make the ball curve left and right, dive "about two feet" and rise—at a time *the riser* was considered impossible. He pitched between his legs, from his knees, behind his back, from center field, second base, blindfolded—with the same result: Few saw it, fewer hit it. In a televised exhibition at Dodger Stadium in 1964, Feigner faced six of the best hitters in baseball: Willy Mays, Willy McCovey, Maury Wills, Harmon Killebrew, Roberto Clemente and Frank Robinson. Pitching from a softball distance of forty-six feet, he struck all of them out in a row—a classic example of the principles of motor learning at work. The hitters were, without question, highly skilled (with years of practice) and possessed exceptional underlying abilities (hand-eye coordination, balance, timing, etc.) They were accustomed to pitches of all shapes and sizes but not to the shorter distance, the larger ball and the faster pitching speed (Feigner was clocked at 112 MPH). The combined differences created a *non-specific* skill. As similar as the tasks seemed, it was like asking a hockey player to bowl. The big hitters couldn't hit Feigner—the skill and natural ability requirements were unique, there was NO transfer of skill from one task to another *and* not enough time to learn the "new."

My track and field instructor at McMaster University set a world record for the 220-yard dash at 20.5 seconds in 1960. Britain's Peter Radford inspired an interest in the sport that has never waned. I've watched many 100-meter finals—from the dominant Russian sprinters, through Canada's single embarrassment (Ben Johnson) to the exploits of Jamaica's Usain Bolt. The great ones fall into one of two categories: those quick off the blocks and the great closers. Quick off the blocks deals with *reaction time* (how quickly one reacts to a stimulus, in this case a gun). Great closers refer to *movement time* (how quickly someone can complete a task). Research on reaction and movement time shows no direct correlation between the two. Some athletes explode off the blocks in a sprint only to lose to someone who has greater movement-time ability. Research also shows no direct correlation between reaction time and movement time *within* the same individual. That is, an increase in reaction-time ability does not enhance movement-time ability in any proportionate way—evidence that practicing one skill or ability is unlikely to enhance another.

I assisted the Douglas High-School baseball team (Parkland, Florida) with their strength training for two seasons. One day, by error, I walked into the office of the football coach who was immersed in a video demonstrating the proper form of a competitive weight-lifting technique and football staple—the power clean. Most coaches (and strength coaches) believe that the power clean is one of the most functional exercises for football by contributing to a lineman's explosive movement on the field—an obvious belief in transfer. From a strength perspective, the power clean may contribute to success in football but from a skill perspective it does not. If the power clean affects explosive movement off the line as much as they believe, then explosive movement off the line must affect the power clean to the same degree. Which means: Players can stop performing the skill of exploding off the line and not lose efficiency because they have been performing power cleans. No coach would bite on that.

The Conclusion—Short and Sweet

The study of Motor Learning reveals two glaring truths:

> **"Specificity" of skill exists; "transfer" of skill does not.**

And what does all this mean? The majority of non-traditional activities currently in vogue in exercise facilities around the country are skill-based. You've been warned.

REFERENCES

1   Johnston, B.D., *System Analysis*, 2008.

2   Rushall, B.S., Pyke, F.S., *Training for Sports and Fitness*. Melbourne, Australia, 1991.

3   Schmidt, R.A., *Motor Learning and Performance: From Principles to Practice*, Human Kinetics, 1991.

4   Sage, G.W., *An Introduction to Motor-Behavior: A Neuropsychological Approach*, 1971.

5   Rushall, B.S., Pyke, F.S., *Training for Sports and Fitness*. Melbourne, Australia, 1991.

6   Rushall, B.S., *Summary of Specificity*, 1992.

CHAPTER 12

···

Functional Training

My college golf coach was accomplished in every sport he tried—gymnastics, tennis, squash, you name it—everything but golf. John Carruthers could shoot in the low seventies on occasion, but occasions were few and far between. Following our first competitive season (1967) he appointed me captain because, in part, I had something he lacked—consistency. He loved to arrange matches against opponents eager to pick our pockets, once challenging two team members at a course where they were club-champion and runner-up respectively. One shot sixty-seven; the other seventy. My seventy-two was no match and John, nowhere to be found.

Coach's passion for the game was unparalleled. His office was stacked floor-to-ceiling with golf magazines. John was susceptible to the written word—had a weakness for golf tips. One day he asked, *"A California pro believes that if you exhale forcefully on your downswing, you'll gain extra yards. What do you think?"* I quietly cleared my throat. On our next outing John featured a polished King-Kong grunt that launched his ball its utmost distance shot after shot. Was it longer? He thought so. To me, it was the same twenty yards ahead.

A second weakness (and I was honored) was his belief in me. He trusted my judgment to the point that he might have stood on his head to hit a ball if I suggested it would improve his game. Don't get me wrong, I have a deep regard for Coach Carruthers to this day.

John's desire to improve parallels the antics of some (and reaction of many) in today's field of exercise. Someone gets a fresh idea, attracts a gathering and is soon recognized as an "expert." Whether the idea is based in fact or fiction, passion carries the day—with one exception. When the passionate Nautilus inventor was asked how he acquired his exercise expertise (*Playboy* magazine, March, 1983), his reply was swift. *"There are no experts in any field. There are some people arrogant enough to call themselves experts; and many people dumb enough to believe them. I quit school in grade four; I'm not an expert in anything."* (This contradicts the perception of the Ph.D.'s who performed research by his side at the University of Florida and called him "a genius in exercise physiology and body mechanics.")

The influence of self-proclaimed experts and, more recently, large corporations on physical trainers and coaches in this country is enormous. Many within earshot simply subscribe despite the fact that the "new" information is based on false premises, fabricated physiology, poor research (if any) and plain lies—as with the latest craze.

"Functional Training" has enjoyed a recent surge since its inception in the 1960's. According to advocate Paul Chek (in *Movement That Matters*), *"Functional training is, basically, any type of exercise that relates directly to the activities you perform in your daily life . . . in other words, functional training is reality-based: Your body mimics everyday movements that you already perform, but want to perform better."* He describes it as *"action-specific, movement-specific or sports-specific training,"* and defines functional as *"commonly used to indicate 'useful,' 'applicable' or something that works."* Some "experts" define it as the duplication of everyday activities without weights (a squat, for example, best helps a person bend to pick something off the floor). Others believe that the movements should be duplicated with added resistance. While a consensus may prove irrelevant, the basic premises of functional training follow:

1. **The body works as a whole** and must be trained as such, using exercises and movement patterns that engage multi-joint systems. Muscle integration produces a better functional outcome and has a greater effect on the general motor program. Isolation, by contrast, is rare and unwarranted in exercise, rehabilitation and strength assessment.

2. ***"Train the movement (skill), not the muscle (strength)."***
    Chek advocates exercises that: ONE, develop skill levels and
    movement patterns; TWO, challenge the nervous system without
    disrupting the motor-learning process (due to complexity); and
    THREE, address the needs of the trainee (determined by a general
    movement evaluation).

3. **Exercise should occur in an unstable environment** to
    activate the body's static stabilization or postural system. The
    support of benches or machines inhibits the body from learning
    balance and stability which results in the pathological loading
    of ligaments and joint instability. Learning can be enhanced by
    practicing high-skill movements and full-body exercises on Swiss
    balls. Balance training on a wobble board, for example, helps
    prevent ankle injury (because the ankle performs exercise in an
    unstable environment). Plyometric training prepares the body for,
    and prevents injury from, high forces. According to Chek, *"Stability
    must always precede force generation."* Force generated by muscle
    contraction produces movement.

4. **Exercises should promote, encourage or replicate
    *"primal movement patterns"*** (general motor abilities that do
    not require special skill): Twisting (to throw a spear), Pulling (to
    return the day's "kill" to the cave), Lunging (to step over a log
    with the "kill" on your shoulders), Bending (to flip food on the fire),
    Squatting (to pick up something) and Pushing (to throw a heavy rock
    off your chest). As a fitness professional, Chek detected a common
    inability to efficiently perform primal patterns at a subconscious
    level. His solution: Enhance the physical impressions made in the
    nervous system by improving skill. His method: Determine patterns
    commonly used, assess their performance and design a functional
    workout that includes Swiss-ball training to correct the problem(s).

5. **Transfer exists between one activity and another.** That is,
    repetition of a movement similar to the target activity (the one you
    are trying to improve) has a positive effect on the performance of
    the target activity. And more: the quality of one action extends to

others—the "explosive" nature of the clean-and-jerk, for example, makes football players more "explosive" on the field.

6. **Abilities can be improved by functional training.** That includes balance, agility, hand/eye coordination, etc.

Now, the bad news . . .

A Critique

The body must be trained as a whole. According to an online definition provided by the BOSU Balance-Trainer Complete Workout System, *"Functional training is purpose driven or intentional training . . . used to expose an individual to integrated movement patterns . . . Functional training encompasses an evolved performance approach that involves the whole body . . . moves away from isolation or single-joint training, to whole body, integrated, multi-joint movement that requires muscle groups to work together."*

"Evolved" should mean "a step forward." Yet, the exclusive use of multi-joint exercises to strengthen movement patterns and correct functional deficiencies is "a step backwards" as Dr. Greg Bradley-Popovich (DPT, MSEP, MS, CSCS, CEI), Director of Clinical Research, NW Spine Management, Rehabilitation and Sports Conditioning, Portland, Oregon, suggests:

"Within a rehabilitative context, functional training may be described as training that mimics elements of the complex movements of daily living. Although I am not opposed to all forms of functional training and believe select exercises can be successfully implemented when used judiciously, the manner in which functional training is commonly implemented, in my view, is flawed. Most commonly, functional training movements are compound (i.e., multi-joint) motions with the underlying logic being that most real-life movements are in fact compound. Herein lies the problem: If only complex motions are used to overload a movement pattern, then the best conditioned muscles in the kinetic chain can accept the brunt of the work. In other words, use of compound movements may do nothing at all to stimulate a weak muscle in the chain because other muscles are permitted

to substitute. As the compensating muscles grow stronger, the strength disparity between the substituting muscles and the weakened muscle(s) may grow greater. Such imbalances may lead to increased biomechanical stress (i.e., wear and tear).

While it is true that a chain is only as strong as its weakest link, this is true of only relatively simple movements. In contrast, gross movements of multiple-body segments may be accomplished by a number of subtly different means—and therefore by a number of different muscles. A prime example of how muscles can compensate is the relationship of the muscles involved in trunk extension: paraspinal lumbar muscles, gluteals, and hamstrings. In patients with chronic low back pain, isolated paraspinal muscle strength is typically diminished. But, any attempt to overload the low back muscles through a supposedly functional task such as lifting weighted boxes may be nullified by compensatory involvement of the hamstrings and gluteals with no meaningful exercise delivered to the low back. And, the small muscles of the low back are the only muscles in a position to finely control motion of individual vertebral segments. Natural muscle synergies such as the cooperative efforts of the aforementioned muscles of truncal extension are truly synergistic only if each contributing muscle pulls its own weight, so to speak.

The lesson to be learned from the number of aberrant muscle substitution pathways is that weak links need to be identified early through isolated analysis and trained in an isolated fashion. Efforts to overload complex movements while ignoring inherent weak links are most often misdirected." [1]

Despite the insistence on multi-joint exercise, Paul Chek believes you should "find the weakness and drill it." But how you can "drill" the weak link in the chain when there is excessive interaction from other muscles and no isolation? To insist on whole-body participation to correct a specific developmental imbalance or weakness is like asking your dentist to drill all of your teeth when the problem is located in one.

The exclusive use of multi-joint exercises is also "a large step backwards" in regard to strength gains. More on that later . . .

2. **Train the movement, not the muscle.** In *Movement That Matters*, Chek states, *"Teaching movement is teaching skill,"* and adds, *"the body knows nothing of muscles, only of movement."* As such he recommends we ***"train the movement, not the muscle."*** His reasoning: Functional exercises score high on a scale of motor complexity (require greater skill than machine exercises) and better enhance overall ability by establishing positive motor "engrams" (physical impressions on nerve tissue that provide a basis for motor memory). According to Chek, Swiss-ball exercises help improve the quality of that impression.

Before it piles too high . . .

- How does Swiss-ball training create or improve general motor engrams when you consider the specificity of each engram (impression) relative to each specific task?
- Being good at one Swiss-ball exercise does not ensure success at another or success at non-Swiss-ball tasks. Motor patterns based on skill are unique and do NOT transfer to other tasks.
- Overall ability is genetically fixed and cannot be "enhanced." Ability allows for the demonstration of specific skills, and consequently, the demonstration of abilities within one's genetic capability. A general motor program dictates natural ability and cannot be altered.
- If the body knows "nothing of muscles," is it unaware that the strength of muscle contraction is the *only* thing that can produce human movement? Not likely.

Chek's point is this: The body integrates contributions from many muscles to accomplish a task. We should, therefore, focus on complex rather than single-joint movements. If single-joint (or machine) exercises are performed to strengthen muscle, then, he suggests, *". . . adequate time must be spent training the muscle to contribute to a functional movement pattern."* In other words, to best apply strength you must skill train—allow the nervous system to put the puzzle together. True, but Chek's method of achieving that goal would roll Arthur over in his grave: *"The integration of full-body participation,"* claims Chek, *"is best accomplished by performing exercise on a Swiss ball"*. The ONLY way to effectively skill train is to practice the skill you want to improve within a *specific* motor program.

Movement and performance depend on two major factors: muscle strength and skill. The result of muscle contraction (the strength system) is the performance of a skill controlled by the central nervous system (the skill system). Contributions by inherited abilities affect the quality of the final product.

Jones believed that training to improve skill and training to improve strength MUST remain apart. Skill training is specific, must PRECISELY mimic the activity or skill one is trying to improve with NO alteration of ANY factor that could influence the practice or performance of the skill, including a change of resistance. Effective skill training requires NO resistance other than that of the implement used in the performance of the skill (tennis racquet, golf club, shot put, etc.). In addition, the intensity of skill training must prevent a high level of fatigue, which could negatively affect the quality of performance (a "fresh" versus "fatigued" effort).

Strength training, on the other hand, is general in its application. A strong triceps will help any movement that involves triceps. In addition, best results from strength training require what Jones called *"outright hard work"*—the use of maximum overload, intensity and fatigue to stimulate change.

The two are at odds. Skill acquisition requires specificity, no resistance, low-to-moderate effort and thrives on brief, frequent training sessions. Strength gain requires no specificity, maximum overload, high levels of intensity and is best acquired by brief, infrequent workouts. Despite the obvious, "functional" advocates insist on training movement patterns against resistance, which compromises both (strength and skill) through belief in three false premises: ONE, that specificity in skill training does not exist; TWO, that skill transfer occurs automatically when you practice an activity similar to (but not exact to) the original skill; and THREE, that a muscle can reach its strength potential through the exclusive use of multi-joint exercises. The first two premises have been proven false by Motor Learning research (as discussed in Chapter 11). The third is a blatant lie and needs no proof.

3. **Exercise should occur in an unstable environment**. Chek references the importance of a system that doesn't exist—the body's static stabilizer or postural system. Every muscle in the body experiences the act of stabilization at one time or another. Muscles have two attachment

points in order to contract: They attach "from somewhere" (origin) and go "to somewhere" (insertion). "Functional" advocates insist that, where possible, muscles should work across both attachments, which is why Chek calls leg-curl machines "useless" because one joint (the knee) is fixed. Yet he fails to acknowledge leg presses and squats (that engage two joints simultaneously) as "functional" exercises; or concede that the movement of some "everyday activities" occurs at one joint only; or admit that what requires a muscle to act as an antagonist in one task may require it to act as a stabilizer or agonist in another.

He also believes that postural dysfunction results in the inability to demonstrate proper function. If so, how does rolling around on a Swiss ball correct the condition? The specific motor pattern of Swiss-ball exercise cannot help the condition of a different motor pattern, in this case, the supposed dysfunction.

An increase in stability (in the functional approach to exercise) requires a focus on highly unstable exercises and full-body movements on a Swiss-ball. Advocates argue that the greater instability provided by—and experienced during—Swiss-ball training promotes stability (and balance) in sports. Non-advocates see it differently. How can the practice of something less stable (than before) *increase* stability in a motor pattern—unless Swiss balls are "magical," as Chek suggests?

Ironically, the only weakness that can be corrected with a Swiss-ball exercise is the skill itself—the proper performance of the exercise on a Swiss ball.

Orthopedic surgeon, Dr. Michael Fulton took the debate a step beyond. In 2005 he received a call from a physical therapist in Iowa and offered her a position in his state-of-the-art rehabilitation facility in Daytona Beach, Florida. She agreed—and things worked well the first year. One morning Fulton spotted several large colored balls and, on further inspection, a variety of colorful tubing with handles. *"First thing,"* he said, *"I pulled out my penknife."* He punctured the balls and cut the tubing which prompted the therapist to resign the next day, claiming she couldn't work with people who were, *"not her kind."* The doctor asked me by phone, *"We're all homo sapiens, aren't we?"* Yes . . . and some are capable of rational thought.

Another word about stability: The body likes to know where it is and where it's supposed to go when we learn skills. It does so through a preparatory hierarchy (*in order*):

1. The body and mind establish proper posture: Head, neck, trunk, spine and other body segments coordinate with foot placement to produce an ideal base of support, if not already established.
2. The large muscle groups closest to the center of the body (hips, thighs, upper back and chest) contract to keep the body balanced relative to the action being performed.
3. The small muscle groups in the peripheral areas contract and work with the basic postural and motor components.

Hence, basic and innate motor skills are taken care of *prior to* the execution of specific tasks. Large muscles contract *first*, followed by small—the process remains constant (regardless of movement speed) and produces an orderly, efficient movement pattern as practiced and determined through the acquired skills. The integration of large and small (muscles) produces one fluid motion of proper position, posture, balance and execution. This *large-to-small* sequential priority of the stabilization process does not sit well with "core" advocates who view "stabilizers" as small muscles that pave the way for large-muscle movement. Chek believes that stability precedes force generation, and it does—but he fails to consider the following:

- Stability and *large-to-small* muscle integration occurs in ANY exercise movement—is NOT limited to "functional" exercises—and should not be deemed crucial to functional improvement.
- The nature of and stability requirements for sport skills, everyday activities and functional training exercises are different. Consequently, functional exercise CANNOT enhance equilibrium and balance in an unlike task any better than traditional exercise.

4. **Exercise should focus on primal movements**. I first thought functional training took us back fifty years, but in light of Chek's caveman analogies, my estimate may have been conservative. "Primal patterns," by his definition, are natural INNATE movement patterns based on ability. Innate means NOT SUBJECT TO CHANGE, yet Chek puts a lot of energy into improving what he calls poor motor engrams. If a person demonstrates

poor ability to complete primal patterns, he or she could have: ONE, a genetic problem; TWO, an injury that affects his or her ability to perform; or THREE, a de-conditioned body (lack of strength and/or flexibility). In the case of the third, proper exercise and activity in general (through a traditional fitness regimen) would prepare the body to better perform the tasks. "Lack of use" causes more problems than poor motor engrams. Weak links within the system must be determined and corrected by balancing the strength, hypertrophy and flexibility of the tissues, not by duplicating primal patterns using highly-unstable, full-body coordination exercises on a Swiss ball or some other useless implement.

And more . . . if the lunge (or any other pattern) is innate (a basic, primitive motor program within our design), it doesn't require practice to improve. Lack of strength and flexibility typically cause problems in movement proficiency . . . not poor, innate motor patterns.

5. Transfer exists between activities. At this level of education you'd think functional advocates would know better, but they don't. In the July/August 2011 issue of *American Fitness* magazine, Angie Miller, MS writes, *". . . simply put, functional training involves training for everyday movement and activity, and applying exercises that transfer to real life."* The skill aspect of exercise WILL NEVER transfer to real life.

The skill acquired through the practice of an exercise remains unique to that exercise. Practice of a machine chest press, for example, increases skill and performance on that machine only. Practice of a free-weight chest press on a bench increases chest-press skill with free weights on a bench. The same with a chest press on a Swiss ball; you eventually master the skill. While none of the skills acquired in one exercise assist the skills acquired in another, the strength gained in any of the presses may increase performance in any of the others. Strength transfers from one activity to another; skill does not.

To illustrate the point, IART founder Brian Johnston suggests trying an agility drill that coaches use with athletes. First, hop laterally (side to side) over a small stool, box or object (under six to eight inches high) for ten to fifteen repetitions. Now, try the same with your ankles tied together and note: The lack of space between your feet alters the motor pattern.

Next, untie your legs and hop with an uneven rhythm (a hop-hop-pause-hop-hop-hop-pause—or any arrhythmic combination). Then, tie your ankles and try it again. The alteration of the timing interferes with what was previously practiced as your mind and body strive to maintain a steady rhythm regardless of the speed of movement. The simple change creates a drastic difference in skill application. Now, consider how removed these lateral hops are to actual athletic events that may require lateral agility in a different environment with different stimuli and a different measure of application. Beyond simple improvement in condition, these agility drills have NO purpose—do not translate to "real life."

Sorry, Angie.

6. Abilities can be improved by functional training. Trainers are often asked to address the following: *"My balance is bad."* My reply is worse, *"General balance cannot be improved."* Balance is a genetically-determined ability formed at an early age and not subject to change. Functional experts disagree. They believe balance can be improved by practice; after all, if balance sensors are activated by practicing Task A, they will improve balance during any task that involves the same sensors. Wrong. The apparent improvement in balance on tasks practiced in a training environment is due to an improvement in skill related to the task at hand. Skill is specific. Abilities, including balance, are general underlying genetic traits that support skill performance. When balance forms an integral part of a skill, it improves ONLY in relation to that skill. It will not improve the balance involved in other skills because the requirements of the new task are specific. As with skill acquisition, balance training does NOT transfer from one task to another—which should direct trainers to select *specific* balance tasks. For example, *to improve the balance required to exit a sofa, bring in the sofa.*

What frequently occurs in the training environment is "customer satisfaction." Trainers take on a balance request because it has been forced upon them by an industry that has developed tools specifically for the purpose. As the client improves the skill of standing on one leg (or on a Bosu ball, balance board, etc.), the trainer delivers the magic words, *"See, you're getting better,"* and everyone lives happily ever after. The implication: Your balance has improved and will be better at ALL tasks that involve balance. But facts don't lie: Your *skill* has improved at the task you practiced, a task in which balance (among other abilities) plays a supporting role; but neither skill nor balance transfer. In the end (and in most cases) the client has mastered a useless skill and is left with the illusion that his general balance has improved. Well-intentioned ignorance converts to customer satisfaction.

Conclusion

My first sports hero, Eddie Feigner faced what he hoped was his last batter. The pitcher of the famous four-man softball team, The King and his Court, had the upper hand—two outs, two strikes on the batter in the bottom of the seventh and a one-run lead on a nine-man All-Star Team. Suddenly, Eddie heard a cry from the umpire, "Time!" The opposing coach took the batter aside, *"He likes to throw the last pitch of the game behind his back. Be ready."* Eddie revved the windmill one last time. His muscular arm rose to its peak then swerved to the rear on the down. The coach was right . . . but too late. The catcher's mitt made its familiar sound and the umpire his, "SteeeRike!" The place exploded. The All-Star bench emptied. The crowd descended on the ump. Eddie headed to a waiting van, ball in hand, and listened as they argued over a pitch he called "The Phantom." *"They thought it was too high,"* he chuckled. Fact ONE: Few could see, let alone hit, any pitch of Feigner's—which ultimately created room for discussion. Fact TWO: Everyone was caught in the frenzy of a high pitch while no one bothered to check the catcher's mitt. Fact THREE: When the smoke cleared, Feigner was halfway to the next town.

Sound familiar? In exercise, everyone gets whipped up about the latest—they *must* try Pilates, functional or performance training—without checking credentials. The fact that everyone is doing it and loves it seems proof enough—which reminds me of what Arthur Jones once said, the best advice concerning functional training. *"If you want to discover something about exercise, write down all the questions, go to a local gym and find the biggest guy there. Ask every question and record every word the man says. Take the information home, do the exact opposite and you'll be one step in the right direction."*

> **. . . to improve the balance required to exit a sofa, bring in the sofa.**

Brian Johnston sums it up best:

"It is ironic that even after a concept is explained in simple terms, so that a child can understand, that well educated, intelligent people will continue to ignore the facts and the common sense arguments put forth in this (his own) critique. They uphold their biases because of politics or ego. They refuse to listen or understand in order to sustain their beliefs, and often to sustain the financial niche they have created for themselves in the marketplace (a niche based on falsehood).

If the reader considers him or herself a student of science, it is vital that the concept of cause and effect be accepted, rather than coincidence. We must uphold that standard before going off half-cocked to accept what we think might be true, based on casual observation or what 'authorities' tell us. Authorities, including Paul Chek, are not always correct, and neither am I, for that matter. We must weigh the evidence relative to what is known and what is fact (and common sense in many instances) and draw our conclusions accordingly." [2]

I've drawn mine.

REFERENCES

[1] Johnston, B.D., *System Analysis*, Bodyworx Publishing, 140, 2001.

[2] Johnston, B.D., *System Analysis*, Bodyworx Publishing, 177, 2001.

CHAPTER 13

Functional Training
Versus
Traditional Training

F unctional exercise trains movement patterns with or without resistance—combines skill and strength training—to produce, according to its advocates, a more "functional" outcome. How wrong they are. From a skill perspective, functional training CANNOT and WILL NOT work. The elements of specificity and transfer inherent in the study of Motor Learning render the claims of skill improvement and transfer impossible, if not fraudulent. And the alleged strength benefits of functional training lead to one conclusion: Why bother?

Arthur Jones viewed a functional outcome his way.

"Human performance is a product of five factors . . . 1) bodily proportions, 2) neurological efficiency, 3) cardiovascular ability, 4) skill, and 5) muscular strength. All of these factors are important . . . but it should be clearly understood that only one factor is actually productive, the other four being supportive in nature.

Ideal bodily proportions for a particular activity may be almost entirely responsible for a championship performance . . . if the other four factors are at least average; but bodily proportions perform no work on their own, their contribution to performance consists of providing the working muscles with an advantage in leverage.

Superior neurological efficiency is also important for a high level of performance . . . but again, it performs no work itself; it merely permits work with a higher than average degree of efficiency.

Cardiovascular ability is an absolute requirement for life itself . . . and a lack of this ability will certainly prevent a high level of performance; yet . . . no amount of cardiovascular ability will perform work. Movement is produced only by the working muscles.

Skill may well be the single most important factor in any activity, but skill cannot perform work. What it does do is provide the working muscles with the ability to work at a higher level of efficiency . . . it channels the force produced by the muscles into a proper direction, and helps to prevent the waste of energy involved in an unskilled performance.

All of the first four factors are important . . . but none of them do the slightest amount of work. The fifth factor is the only one that is actually productive . . . all of the others help, but only the muscles perform work.

When the previously mentioned points are understood, it becomes obvious that the five factors should be divided into two categories . . . four supportive factors in one category . . . and one productive factor in the other category.

And . . . the same five factors should also be divided into two other categories, since two of the five factors are determined by genetics and three factors can be improved. So our attention and efforts should be restricted to the three factors that can be improved.

Absolutely nothing can be done to improve either bodily proportions or neurological efficiency. We must do the best we can with what we have . . . these factors are either good or bad, but are outside our realm of control in any case.

But we can do something about the other three factors . . . these can be improved, and should be. At this point in the history of sports, a very high percentage of training is devoted to the improvement of skill . . . and it should be, since skill is probably the single most important factor in most activities. Cardiovascular ability is also given a great deal of attention . . .

and again, it should be, since a lack of at least adequate cardiovascular ability will certainly limit performance.

In a sense, cardiovascular ability is linked very closely to skill . . . since skill results only from the practice of a particular activity, which activity will also help to produce the required level of cardiovascular fitness. Skill in basketball, for example, is produced only by playing basketball . . . and the level of cardiovascular ability required for basketball is produced by the same training.

Additionally, most athletes also practice some form of training that is intended only for the purpose of increasing cardiovascular . . . so in most sports cardiovascular ability is given the degree of attention that it deserves.

Thus, in practice, two of our three improvable factors are already receiving the attention they require . . . while one improvable factor remains largely neglected. And, as it happens, the neglected factor just happens to be the only actually productive factor on the list . . . the only factor capable of producing movement, the only factor able to perform work. Muscular strength is the neglected factor." [1]

Jones also believed (from Chapter 3) that Proper Strength Training was capable of producing five benefits: Improvements in strength, flexibility, cardiovascular condition, body composition and injury protection. Let's examine the contribution(s) of "Functional Training" to each.

A. Strength

The focus on movement patterns rather than the muscles that produce them results in poor strength gains for several reasons: ONE, inadequate resistance; TWO, the exclusive use of "integrative," multi-joint or compound movements; and THREE, low levels of intensity.

Inadequate Resistance

The go-to tools of functional training are latex bands, bodyweight, pulleys and (to a lesser extent) free weights. *"The freedom of movement* (provided by these choices)," they say, *"is necessary to exercise the body through unlimited planes and directions."* In other words, machines restrict the path of movement during exercise. At the same time, functional advocates fail to acknowledge that their choices ignore a factor of far greater importance—quality of resistance.

Latex bands, for example, are throwbacks from rehab centers: They "feel" different than free weights because they are. During pushing and pulling exercises, bands provide less resistance at the start of the movement (in extension) and more at the end (in contraction)—which is, at least, a change in the right direction. They do, however, fail to deliver a sufficient overload in ANY position—exercises are rarely hard enough to stimulate change—and progress is difficult to measure.

Despite its recent popularity, bodyweight is NOT the best choice of resistance. In high-school PE class, Coach never unveiled the rusty set of barbells stuffed in the closet by the boy's locker room. He used chin-ups, push-ups and other bodyweight exercises. Chin-ups required the use of full weight, while push-ups required a lesser percentage and were not as difficult. Some exercises were tough but it didn't take long to discover that bodyweight did NOT compare to barbells, and later, that barbells did NOT compare to the overload provided by machines.

In general, pulleys and free-weights are better choices than bodyweight and bands but they too fail to deliver a direct resistance and one that varies with the muscle's needs through the range of motion. Few seem concerned: *Why use a quality resistance when you can use something less?*

The same applies to quantity.

The supposed advantage of movement-pattern training, full-body participation and multi-tasking in unstable environments (all functional-training concepts) adversely affects the *quantity* of resistance you can safely use. If you normally arm-curl eighty pounds for ten repetitions, for example, and suddenly find yourself perched on an air-filled balance pad, you can no longer use eighty. Take a leg away and you must further reduce the load. Stand on a tightrope over Niagara Falls while you sing "God Save The Queen" . . . you get the point: More complex tasks require less resistance. The good news:

According to Barnum & Bailey®, you are now more "functional." The bad: The strength potential of your biceps (in the example above) will forever elude.

Ten years ago, Jim Flanagan's advice on the purchase of exercise machines for a new gym was clear: *"Whatever you do,"* said the MedX general manager, *"avoid the Cybex 'Dual Axis' line. The movement arms skate freely . . . and are dangerous as hell."* A year later I used three of the machines while on vacation and Jim was right. Without the skill to control the movement arm, the devices were dangerous. I had to reduce the resistance to "feel" safe. Yet, what functional trainers hail a plus (that reduced stability forces involvement of "stabilizers" to support working muscles), Arthur Jones hailed a minus. *"The only thing likely to happen,"* he said, *"is injury to the 'balancing' muscles."* Ironically, the warning label on the "Dual-Axis" machines states: **Arms move in paths directed by user. Incorrect path can cause injury. Movement must be controlled in proper path.** The machines provide freedom of choice, yet manufacturers pray you choose a path they are unwilling to define. I wouldn't be concerned. From *every* path, the logic behind instability training for strength makes no sense: *Why use a resistance high enough to stimulate change when you can use less and stimulate nothing?*

Integrative Exercise

According to functional experts, exercise should be "integrative"—involve several joints. This compound approach activates more muscle mass to better shock the system from both strength and cardiovascular perspectives (more muscle work demands a greater heart response). But, it has a negative side. When movement occurs over several joints, the weak link in the chain is either A) overloaded, which results in one of two things: Muscle growth stimulation (a good thing) or injury (a bad thing), or B) bypassed, which does nothing to strengthen the weakness. More often than not, the stronger muscles compensate for the weak and don't allow them to work. Nonetheless, functional training evaluations attempt to identify muscle weakness based on movement screens. Once identified, multi-joint exercises are chosen (according to Paul Chek) to "hammer the weakness." How can you "hammer the weakness" by taking a general stab at a specific problem? You can't strengthen front-thigh muscles to their maximum, for example, without using a leg-extension machine. Yet, functional trainers consider the leg-extension machine "useless" because it isolates and because it is a machine—a cryin' shame when what they advocate—compound exercise—does NOT allow ANY muscle to EVER reach its strength potential.

Another limitation: Multi-joint exercise does not require the muscles involved to move through a full range of motion and, thus, fails to provide full-range exercise. When a muscle cannot reach a position of full contraction where all of its fibers are potentially involved, maximum strength gains are impossible. When a muscle fails to reach full extension, flexibility increases are equally impossible.

Intensity

Two ingredients are required to produce best results from strength training: good form and high levels of intensity. If work intensity does not reach a high percentage of effort required to trigger change, stimulation will not occur. No intensity = No stimulation = No change. Despite the obvious, functional trainers avoid high intensity (working muscles to failure) at all cost to not *"overtax the nervous system."* My first glimpse of functional exercise left me puzzled. Why would anyone exercise on the floor with no resistance in a gym full of great tools—and eagerly pay for what they once rejected in high school? It made no sense.

Despite their propensity to avoid intense efforts, functional advocates believe that movement-training *enhances* strength. Research suggests otherwise:

"Carlile and Carlile (1961) reported that Australian swimmers trained with weight exercises prior to commencing hard swimming training in preparation for an Olympic Games. During the swimming training, no weight training was performed. After 10 weeks of swimming training that produced over-trained states, thereby attesting to the intensity of the training load, it was found that strength gains that had previously been achieved prior to swimming had regressed back to untrained levels." [2]

If strength is the ONLY productive factor in human performance—and the most neglected as Jones believed—it will remain neglected after the proper application of functional exercise. The strength contribution of functional training to human performance is sub-standard at best.

B. Flexibility

As with all cardiovascular training, the "multi-joint" exercise frenzy of functional training does not allow muscles to reach full extension where stretching can occur. This promotes partial-range movement and flexibility loss. On the other hand, traditional strength training often takes muscles to positions where a stretch can occur . . . but that's not enough. There must be adequate resistance in that position—a back force pushing against the muscle—to trigger the proper response. The resistance provided by free-weight exercises rarely meets that criterion, but a machine with a proper cam provides resistance in full-extension and allows muscle/joint systems to reach the limit of their range of motion. Properly performed, exercise machines *increase* flexibility with built-in progress: An increase in resistance exposes muscles to greater force in extension, increasing the potential for stretch. On the other hand, well-performed functional exercise CANNOT increase flexibility, unless a supplemental stretching program is implemented. Ironically, many bodybuilders are flexible *because of* their training while many functional advocates are flexible (if they are) *in spite of* theirs.

C. Cardiovascular Condition

The difference between cardiovascular benefits gained through traditional versus functional training is slight. On the one hand, when exercise is performed with no rest between efforts, the intensity and quality of resistance favors traditional training: Non-stop hard work with superior resistance elicits a high cardiovascular demand. On the other, the volume of muscle mass involved in multi-joint exercise favors functional training.

Ironically, many bodybuilders are flexible *because of* their training while many functional advocates are flexible (if they are) *in spite of* theirs.

For the record, the greatest cardiovascular result in the history of exercise was produced during "Project Total Conditioning," an experiment at the US Military Academy in West Point (1975) described in the chapter that follows. The strength-training program, designed and orchestrated by Arthur Jones, produced "incredible" cardiovascular results measured by a team of aerobic experts. Shocking to some and insulting to others, members of the football team created the results as they sat on machines.

D. Body Composition

Functional training makes a poor contribution to the loss of body fat because it fails to stimulate significant muscle mass. Muscles grow when stimulated to increase in strength and the most efficient way to reduce body fat is to increase muscle mass—a concept foreign to a system that focuses on movement. Because the force of muscle contraction is the ONLY factor that PRODUCES movement, you'd think "functional" advocates would pay more attention to the strength of the tools they use. As a result, the effect of their training—properly performed—is greater on the cardiovascular system than the muscle system, leaving trainees with body-composition results similar to those produced by cardiovascular activity—*indiscriminate* weight loss. Bodyweight lost through participation in functional exercise comes from muscle, organ and fat tissue. Loss of the first two is undesirable.

Muscle-mass increase through strength training provides body-composition advantages. The body not only burns calories during the activity that stimulates the strength change but continues to burn calories during rest—a "double reducing effect" that is absent with both cardiovascular and functional training.

E. Injury Prevention/Protection

Injury is a simple game of numbers. How strong is the structure? How much force is applied to it? If the numbers on one side outweigh the numbers on the other at the moment of truth, the result will be one of two things: injury or no injury. Injury prevention, for the most part, is dependent on the strength of muscles, connective tissue and bones that comprise the joint—not on skill. Even highly-skilled athletes suffer injury when their numbers aren't right.

"Functional" advocates stress the importance of strong joint stabilizers but give little or no credit to the strength of the large muscles that surround the joint—strength that can only be optimized through the use of isolated exercise and maximum resistance. They also ignore the fact that many injuries are caused by the application of excess force to a muscle/joint system while it operates in an unstable environment. Their solution: Operate in a different unstable environment to prepare for the real world: *"Balance on a wobble board to prevent injury to ankles;" "Train with a high-force modality (like plyometrics) to prepare the body for high forces."* Something's missing. Since each skill is unique and the number of possible motor patterns countless, every conceivable angle and body position would have to be trained to establish strength in all the pathways necessary to prevent injury. Yet, only a handful of specific Swiss-ball and other functional exercises are included in any one program. Hence, functional exercises are no more beneficial for injury prevention than more stable free-weight or machine exercises.

Paul Chek believes that injury is more a function of *"faulty movement patterns"* than weak structural support. He recommends avoiding fixed patterns during exercise (machines that restrict movement to a single path) but fails to acknowledge that free-weight and functional exercises have their own fixed patterns. A heavy bench press that moves "off path," for example, may quickly reveal the thickness of your skull. Furthermore, if a faulty movement pattern places the body into positions that improperly stress the muscles, how does traditional exercise (with free weights or machines) fortify faulty patterns that may lead to injury? All exercise abides by joint/muscle movement requirements. What is faulty about a machine curl that requires the elbow joint to flex?

A Master functional trainer recently lectured in our facility. His promotional flyer, **"Are You Training Movement or Muscle?"** mentioned the following: *"How often have you heard of the guy who strengthens his muscles in the traditional way only to find that when he bends over, he pulls out his back?"* The assumption is misleading. The man did not injure himself because of a faulty movement pattern—failure to train the movement of bending over. He injured it because the forces involved in bending exceeded the strength of his muscle/joint system at that moment.

The assumption ignores another fact. Functional training, like traditional training, has NO effect on the strength of the lumbar spine. Research has shown that isolated exercise on a highly specific machine is the ONLY meaningful way to strengthen the muscles that extend the torso. Unfortunately, both isolation and the use of machines are concepts foreign to functional exercise.

Added strength protects you from injury; added skill through unrelated movement-training does not. And that applies to sports, activities of daily living and . . .

Rehabilitation

Functional trainers believe that the application of their methodology has great value in rehabilitation, where specific needs of agility, power, strength and balance can be addressed. Yet, they fail to consider: ONE, that the measure and application of balance, agility or any other ability is different from one task to another; TWO, that transfer of abilities from one movement pattern to another is impossible; and THREE, that general abilities such as balance and agility are genetically fixed and not subject to change. They can only be demonstrated through specific practiced skills.

Low-Back Rehabilitation

If you walked into a clinic with a biceps problem and the doctor urged you to *"strengthen your triceps,"* you might leave. Yet, we accept the same advice with low backs. *"Strengthen your abs"* has become the gold standard in back care—that strong abdominals support the spine from the anterior and establish a dynamic interrelationship with the muscles of the low back. Arthur Jones disagreed.

After testing the isolated strength of the muscles that extend the lumbar spine in approximately 10,000 subjects, he concluded that abdominal strength had NOTHING to do with back pain. *"Ninety-nine point nine, nine percent (99.99%) of the people on the planet,"* he stated, *"are walking around in a state of chronic disuse atrophy. They have never used those muscles."*

When many of the same subjects were exposed to "valid" exercise, the unused muscles gained strength at a rate that Dr. Michael Pollock (University of Florida) could not believe but had to—his team measured them. Jones called the device that provided the exercise, the MedX Lumbar Extension machine, *"the closest thing to a miracle I have ever seen"*—and Arthur did NOT believe in miracles. "He invented the machine," you say. "What do you expect?" If nothing else, Jones was honest to a fault.

If something else, he spent years in the large-animal business and had an extensive collection of rhinos, snakes, elephants and reptiles at his home in Ocala, Florida. He called a 17½-foot Australian brute (one of 1,400), "the world's largest crocodile." And it may have been . . . but for this: Paul Chek's claim of being an expert in low-back rehabilitation may well be the largest "croc" in the world.

"Rehab on the back-extension machine," says Chek (with no reference to MedX), *"is like selling part of the Brooklyn Bridge."* After all, a machine that guides the load reduces the need to *"recruit the body's own intrinsic and extrinsic stabilizers."* His mantra: Swiss-ball exercise. Mine: *Good luck . . .*

- The stability and balance requirements to stand, walk or perform an activity are not the same as the stability and balance requirements of any Swiss-ball exercise. Good balance and stability at one task does not guarantee equal or better performance at another.
- If the need to balance and coordinate is reduced or eliminated from an exercise, greater effort and attention can be forwarded to the working muscles rather than on the act of balancing or stabilization. Increased emphasis on fewer tasks may result in a greater inroad per unit of time and superior muscle stimulation. Increased muscle tissue around joints enhances stability, performance and the ability to exert and resist force.
- If balance and stability are altered through injury as to affect proper posture and balance in sports or activities of daily living, would unstable exercise on a Swiss ball be possible or safe?

> **Added strength protects you from injury; added skill through unrelated movement-training does not.**

The prime function of low-back muscles is spinal extension through a range of motion of seventy-two degrees. They do not work optimally unless sufficiently isolated. When the low-back muscles increase in size and strength and are proportionately strong throughout that range (conform to a *normal* strength curve), the stability of the spine as well as the general function of the individual improves.

According to a decade of research at the University of Florida, this status can ONLY be achieved through the extreme isolation offered by the proper use of a machine that prohibits pelvic rotation (see Chapter 18). Full-body integration (as advocated by functional trainers) has NO effect on the strength of the muscles that extend the spine but can negatively affect pain perception. When the large hip muscles become involved (due to pelvic rotation), they ALONE receive the strength benefit but often overload the smaller spinal muscles in the process. Fortunately, the overload parameters of Swiss-ball training are so poor that they are not likely to produce injury or stimulate change. Which makes it clear: *The stability increase claimed by the acquisition of skill in performing functional exercise is different than—and inferior to—the stability acquired through stronger muscles.*

Plyometric, balance and Swiss-ball exercises have never been properly isolated, tested and compared to more traditional protocols. Paul Chek denounces low-back rehabilitation with machines yet ignores the science and success behind the MedX device—for good reason. Clinical trials of *Swiss-balls vs. MedX* would make his opinion resemble the east end of a horse going west.

Swiss-ball training will not likely hurt your low back . . . nor, *in any way*, help it.

Swiss-ball training will not likely hurt your low back...nor, *in any way*, help it.

Conclusion

The term "Functional Training" is deceptive. It CANNOT help trainees reach their functional potential:

FIRST, it minimizes the role of the only productive factor in performance—strength. Arthur Jones trained some of the world's best athletes in Lake Helen, Florida and believed that few, if any, had enough strength or muscle to be anywhere near their potential. *"Short of checkers and chess,"* he said, *"a stronger athlete is a better athlete."* Functional training's approach to strength prevents athletes from *ever* reaching that potential.

SECOND, unless stretching is added, the exclusive use of multi-joint exercises promotes flexibility loss. Partial-range movements do NOT allow muscles to reach positions where stretching can occur.

THIRD, functional training can trigger a high cardiovascular response (one of three improvable factors in human performance) but it is rarely performed with little or no rest between exercises.

FOURTH, the best way to improve the body's muscle-mass/body-fat ratio is to make muscles stronger—of little concern to functional trainers.

FIFTH, strength prevents injury. Joints anchored by strong muscles decrease the chance of injury. Properly trained, a stronger body is one that is leaner, more flexible, uses oxygen more efficiently and better protects itself from external forces.

SIX, with NO transfer, functional training increases skill ONLY in the movement patterns (or exercises) practiced: Practice a wood-chop movement and you get better at a wood-chop; a bench press, you get better at a bench press. The skill gained by practicing either (a bench press or wood-chop) has NO effect on improving the performance of any other activity. On the other hand, the strength gained by practicing either is applicable to ALL skills that involve those muscle groups. Skill (one of three improvable factors in human performance) CANNOT transfer to other activities; strength CAN . . . but the "functional" approach to strength is dismal.

SEVEN, general balance CANNOT improve. Balance specific to a task CAN—as skill improves—but the improvement does NOT transfer to other activities. To improve skill and/or balance in scaling a flight of stairs, strengthen the muscles to be used and then practice scaling the stairs—the same flight.

True lunacy is confirmed by the number of organizations circumventing the globe to dispense the wisdom of functional training. The NASM (National Academy of Sports Medicine), as one example, conducts a functional analysis through the performance of what they call an "overhead squat." From that they determine the direction of the program, starting with correctional exercises. Once the body has balanced strength (however they determine that) and stability (however they determine that), they initiate a program of strength training that is all over the map. To this point and despite philosophical inconsistencies, the program follows what they believe is "a safe, logical path to functional progression."

Then, from the midst of their poetic bliss, they recommend the closest thing to athletic suicide, "plyometrics." Their rationale: The SAID principle (Specific Adaptation to Imposed Demand) which states you must prepare the body for what it will encounter—including impact. Arthur Jones once listened to a self-proclaimed expert denounce the impact of running only to replace it with what he called *"a safe alternative,"* jump squats (a plyometric staple). If the impact forces involved in running are 4-5 times your bodyweight, those involved in jump squats may be 4-5 times higher yet. The extreme forces encountered during plyometric exercise are well documented and advocates either have their collective heads buried deep in "tradition" (such as the NFL) or are plain stupid. In light of their take on plyometric training alone, you should question *everything* proposed by "functional" experts.

At the moment, no one questions a thing.

To Those Who Believe

The worldwide sales pitch for functional training has proven effective. Many athletes swear that their performance has improved as a result of adopting functional training, despite the fact that benefits are limited to an increase in cardiovascular condition (when exercises are performed in rapid sequence) and to the acquisition of unrelated skills. Yet, the claims made by these advocates extend to ANY form of exercise: An overload, within individual tolerance, can produce a benefit. The different challenge of functional exercise might motivate those with a history of exercise to work hard and produce a greater net effect that spills over into their skill training. The claims are further confused by the fact that many trainees practice traditional exercise, skill training and functional training at the same time. In like manner, rehab patients who believe that functional training played a major role in their recovery, also used pills, modalities, stretching or hybrid treatments to confuse the issue.

The above skepticism does little to dampen the spirit of "functional" advocates. *"It really does not matter,"* claims Paul Chek, *"how strong anyone is on a machine exercise . . . there is a VERY POOR correlation between strength during a supported lift (such as a bench press or Smith squat) and any functional task such as breaking through the line in football, controlling an opponent in wrestling or making it through a slalom course in water or on snow."* To prove his point, he developed a *Standing Single-Leg Cable Push Test* that consisted of balancing on one leg and pushing a shoulder-high cable handle straight forward with the opposite arm as if throwing a punch—using 30% of one's 1RM bench-press weight. Athletes who trained with "non-functional" exercise, according to Chek, performed poorly on the test while those with a background in Olympic lifting, martial arts, wrestling, dance or other "functional" exercise systems did best—with NO SPECIFIC TRAINING AT ALL (no test practice).

Great observation, but his test and logic are flawed:

1. *The ability to lift weight in any manner has to do with muscle mass (and its potential for force production), innate ability and the proficiency acquired through the skills of each movement. A muscular traditional-exercise trainee would lift a greater weight in the bench press than a less-muscular functional trainee who does not practice the bench press. A well-developed 200 pound man who can press 400 pounds would use 120 pounds in Chek's test (30% of 400 = 120 pounds) while a 160-pound man who presses 160 pounds will use forty-eight pounds (30% of 160 = 48 pounds).*

The fairness of the test is equivalent to a bodybuilder challenging a functional trainee to an arm curl with a barbell.

2. From a skill perspective, the "bodybuilder" is at a disadvantage because he lacks the skill involved in the balance/push test, especially if the functional trainee practiced the skill (which Chek claims did NOT happen).

3. The innate abilities of the Olympic lifters, martial-arts subjects, wrestlers and dancers may have been superior to those of the traditional-trained subjects who took the test. These genetically-superior abilities may have attracted the athletes to their activity of choice in the first place.

4. Chek's observation flies in the face of decades of research that: ONE, negate the transfer of one skill to another; and TWO, demonstrate that the ability to perform one activity has no correlation to the ability to perform another. Where's his data?

5. His claim that *"motor patterns developed by supported exercises (benches and machines) do not carry over well to standing exercises"* fails to mention that there is NO carryover from one standing exercise to another standing exercise; NO carryover from specific standing exercises to sport tasks (or activities of daily living) that do not require the *exact* same mechanics; and a "VERY POOR correlation between strength gained during Swiss-ball exercises and breaking through the line in football, controlling an opponent in wrestling, etc . . ."

The Value of Increased Muscle

The field of exercise has been inundated with "functional" trainers, many of whom are unaware of the simplicity of what they are trying to accomplish. An increase in performance as it relates to muscle function requires one of two things (or both):

- **First, an increase in skill.** The continual practice of an exercise (or movement) produces greater lifting proficiency (or skill). The establishment of neuromuscular patterns and the accompanying mental integration through practice enhance the ability to lift greater weights or better perform a task.
- **Second, an increase in strength or lean muscle mass.** Muscle gained through strength training increases joint stability and the ability to generate and resist force. This architectural change in tissue can be stimulated by the use of free weights, bodyweight exercise, machines and Swiss-ball exercise—but is NOT exclusive to Swiss-ball and other so-called "functional training" exercises.

Time and again, Chek acknowledges that bodybuilding exercises are best for hypertrophy but ignores the benefit of hypertrophy to meet the goal of improved function. Increased lean muscle tissue results in greater force production (strength) and joint stability (resistance to force). On his Swiss-ball video series, he states that functional training exercises are superior (to traditional exercises) since they create greater stabilization, require far greater skill and, as a result, affect more muscle (based on quantity, not quality of effort per unit). But he fails to consider several important points: ONE, the magnitude of overload with functional training is often insufficient to produce muscle growth; and TWO, functional training and Swiss-ball exercises are not unique to the integration of many muscles. A simple bench press involves the integration of triceps, shoulders and pectorals for control. A wide stance maintains balance on the bench while thighs, calves, abdominals, rotator cuffs and the spine work to stabilize the movement. Is this not "neuromuscular integration?"

According to Chek, it is not. *"If you had to rate bodybuilding exercises for their average level of motor complexity on a scale of 10, 10 being very complex,"* he states, *"then a score of 1-4 would be fair."* Nice speech, especially when the relationship between the value of a highly complex exercise and functional increase has *never* been established—not if we take into account the individuality of skills and abilities within each task.

If I had to rate functional versus traditional exercises for their average level of contribution to increased function on a scale of 10, 10 being the highest, my scores would also be "fair," as follows:

Contribution to:	Functional Exercise	Traditional Exercise
Skill	0	0
Strength	1-4	10
Flexibility	0	7-10
Cardiovascular Condition	7-10	8-10
Body Composition	1-3	8-10
Injury Prevention	1-4	10

It would be fair to say that, compared to traditional means, movement-pattern training is a joke—yet the experts have the audacity to call it "functional."

I stood on the par-three eighth tee of the Olde Mill Golf Club in Laurel Fork, Virginia in 1974. A ten-year-old boy I caught up to during play decided to let me through. The hole demanded a carry of 188 yards over a rugged ravine to a shallow green. I considered two clubs and made the critical selection. The ball flew high and straight, descending on a line just left of the pin. As I posed to admire my work, the ball soared deep into the jagged ravine beyond the green. When the smoke cleared, the kid spoke up, *"Nice shot, Mister. You just got a bad result."*

And so it is with those who choose functional training as their ticket to the Promised Land. You can do everything right along the way and ultimately end with "a bad result."

Why bother?

It would be fair to say that, compared to traditional means, movement-pattern training is a joke, yet the experts have the audacity to call it "functional."

REFERENCES

[1] Jones, A., "Improving Functional Ability in any Sport," Peterson, J.A., Ph.D., (editor), *Total Fitness: The Nautilus Way,* Leisure Press, 8: 83-85, 1978.

[2] Rushall, B.S., Pyke, F.S., *Training for Sports and Fitness.* Melbourne, Australia: Macmillan of Australia, 1991.

CHAPTER 14

··

REAL Functional Training

I f "functional" means that something "works," it follows that functional training is training "that works." Arthur Jones spent a lifetime examining how things worked and built things that did—a machine gun at age eleven, a non-nuclear submarine at fourteen, a vibration-free camera mount for filming from moving platforms (in his case, from vehicles pursuing wild animals), anamorphic lens systems for motion-picture work, exercise machine prototypes, a protocol that addressed the lagging development of his torso and a lumbar machine nominated for a Nobel Prize in medicine. Each Nautilus® machine represented approximately seven years of development; his MedX® medical tools, between fourteen and twenty. Jones refused to market a product that did not meet his high standards or conform to the phrase, *"Function dictates design."* It had to work—and did, as Robert Glenn (Post-Production Supervisor for *Daktari*) suggested, *". . . if he says that his new machines work, then they work better than he says."*

Arthur's singular focus did not prevent him from seeing the big picture. He believed there were many ways to get the job done with exercise but that some were better than others. In the early days he helped bodybuilders achieve size and strength goals (and athletes reach performance potentials) by steering them in a logical direction. *"You can swim to Hawaii,"* he said to those taking the long route, *"or take a jet."* His tools and system provided the air fare.

Jones' entrance into the field was aimed at finding the truth. *"I tell the truth,"* he said, *"and it shocks people. I am against fraud, against deception."* That's where the problem began—he made people squirm.

His quote, *"Athletes are born, not made,"* for example, was tough to swallow when you were training one. He believed that approximately 80% of one's ability to excel in a sport—to run fast or jump high—was genetically determined. The remainder was in the hands of the athlete and his or her support team—the physical and psychological preparation, skill training, strategy and coaching—things that remain open to interpretation . . .

My business partner in Venezuela was the National Water-Ski Coach; his wife, a seven-year undefeated world-champion in trick skiing. From 1972-1979, Maria Victoria Carrasco competed in forty-four international competitions and retired undefeated. Bad enough that her ski facility was home-made; she performed NO strength training during her reign. In contrast, her younger sister, Ana Maria, worked out religiously in my facility for ten years and held the world trick-ski record during that time. In 1988, Ana was overall world-champion (trick, slalom and jump). Two champions: one trained hard, the other not at all. Maria Victoria probably never reached her potential but it may not have mattered: She was good enough to beat the world with an overdose of favorable genes.

So it was with another client, ninth-round draft-pick, Reed Bohovich. In the summer of 1962 the offensive guard from Lehigh University received a welcome letter and starting-kit from the New York Giants before pre-season training. The kit included a plastic bag which housed an "isometric rope" and instruction sheet. At twenty, the youngest ever to play in the NFL was expected to report to camp "in excellent physical condition." Football had yet to discover barbells. Today, conditioning with an isometric rope wouldn't land a job at the peanut stand. Reed went on to a brief career with the Giants.

I experienced early success in a sport that, combined with a career in training, led to the conditioning of competitive golfers. The challenge began in Caracas when I was asked to prepare Venezuela's male and female teams for the World Team-Amateur Championship in 1988. At the time, I had a 25-machine Nautilus facility, Jones' philosophical approach to strength training for sports, knowledge of golf, an eight-year business reputation and six months to train the athletes. The approach was simple: strengthen the muscles used in golf—then plug the "new and improved" tools into the swing. Both teams performed better than expected but the process wasn't easy. Golfers fear that strength training will negatively affect skill and generally measure progress by their latest score.

A decade later I was hired by a classmate from the MedX Certification Program at the University of Florida to assist in the development of a golf/fitness program in Jupiter, Florida. His facility was well-equipped: four $60,000 MedX medical machines—Lumbar Extension, Torso Rotation, Cervical Extension and Cervical Rotation—and a full line of MedX exercise tools. Three of us designed a program that became a sensation. We analyzed the golf swing with a $40,000 computerized system, matched errors to cures (a sixteen-page matrix) and applied the remedy using strength, functional and stretching exercises. I conducted the strength training while physical therapist, Jessica Parnevik managed the functional end. The program drew the likes of Jack Nicklaus, Jesper Parnevik, Per-Ulrik Johansson, Betsy King, more than a dozen LPGA professionals and a host of locals. Guests flew in from the PGA Tour®, the Champions Tour® and The Golf Channel®. The placed rocked until upper-management conflict led to its demise.

In 2010 another facility where I worked took it a step further by introducing the "Holy Grail" of golf fitness, the Titleist Performance Institute® program. They hired a master TPI trainer, certified two others and prepped the membership—but things fizzled. The master instructor proved inept and one of the trainers suffered an unrelated injury. I thought it would eventually fail for another reason: TPI has its roots in functional training. The studio set of *Golf Fitness Academy* (TV's version of functional exercise sponsored by Titleist®) has wall-to-wall pulleys and playground toys—no machines and few free-weights. All exercise remedies are multi-joint and the hosts believe in transfer. Their saving grace—mass marketing—has brainwashed the world of golf and the clamor for TPI trainers has created a waiting list. How do they measure progress? The same way it was measured in Caracas and Jupiter—"How'd you play today?" Its popularity thrives on the lingering fear that traditional strength training will "screw up" a golf swing or is simply, "not enough." Its beauty: TPI training doesn't *look* traditional and is designed by people who *know* the game, not the dumb trainer at the corner. Its weakness: The program is nothing more than functional training—from analysis to execution—and its benefits remain few: cardiovascular gains (when rest between exercise is minimal) and little to no improvement in skill, flexibility, strength, injury protection or body composition. TPI training CANNOT and WILL NOT meet the expectations of golfers, unless they are low.

Training to reach one's functional potential is not as complicated as some would have you believe . . .

In 1972 Bill Bradford was relieved of his duties as football coach at Deland High School in Florida. Impressed by the results Arthur Jones had produced with *negative-only* exercise in the "Quonset Hut," a makeshift facility behind the school used to train athletes visiting Nautilus Sports/Medical Industries in nearby Lake Helen, he decided to start a weightlifting team. *"At the time,"* said Jones, *"I doubt that he (Bradford) really knew the difference between a barbell and a palm tree, but he was not stupid."* The plan was simple: Build raw strength through the exclusive use of negative exercise (*lowering* rather than *lifting* weights) and practice the lifting techniques required in competition. The execution was equally simple: *"Two weekly workouts, only one set of each exercise, from six to eight repetitions in each set."* The rest is in the books. With no prior history in the sport, Bradford's team went undefeated and untied for seven consecutive years. The approach—to strengthen muscles used in the sport and then practice the sport—was a far cry from today's mega-programs. Coach Bradford *was* smart: He quit while he was ahead. His successor started losing because, according to Jones, *". . . he went back to using conventional methods,"* then added, *"And having been regularly trounced by Bradford's team for seven years, how many other coaches adopted his training method? None. Why not? Damned if I know; but I do know that it is impossible to explain insanity."* The simplicity of the approach was functional training at its best . . .

. . . until Jones stepped it up a notch.

Project Total Conditioning

In 1975 Arthur sold a set of Nautilus machines to the United States Military Academy (West Point, N.Y.) and agreed to a joint venture as described by Captain James A. Peterson, Associate Professor of Physical Education: *"The study (Project Total Conditioning) was designed to provide USMA with the institutional knowledge of how to properly use its Nautilus equipment; to examine the elative effectiveness of different methods of strength training; and finally, (and perhaps, most importantly) to identify the consequences of a short duration, high intensity strength training program."* Peterson designed and directed the study, and claimed, *". . . every effort was made to make 'Project Total Conditioning' the most productive and inclusive field research endeavor ever undertaken in the area of strength training."* [1] It was. Jones would have it no other way.

Part of the project involved the preparation of some of the football team for the upcoming season. At the time the team was practicing twice a day, running two miles on the track (for time) and performing an *unsupervised* circuit of strength training three times per week. The plan was to train a fraction of the players with ONE modification—a *supervised* circuit of strength training using Nautilus machines. Fifty-three cadets were divided into three groups: a Nautilus-Only group (twenty-one), a Control group (sixteen) and a Neck-Only group (sixteen) to verify the effectiveness of prototype neck machines. The Nautilus-Only group, reduced to nineteen by illness and a single football injury, was allocated a two-week trial period to minimize the effect of motor learning. During the trial (and the study) they performed one set of eight to twelve repetitions to muscle failure on ten Nautilus machines three times per week. At the end of the two-week trial Captain Peterson and his staff performed the *initial* testing—strength, flexibility, body composition, etc. Jones contacted the world's foremost expert, Dr. Kenneth Cooper (Dallas, Texas), to test and measure cardiovascular results. When Cooper's team arrived Jones left town and never shook a hand. He did not want results to appear *influenced* in any way.

The procedures for training were *"explicitly objective and precisely controlled"* but the training itself was brutal—a non-stop circuit of high-intensity exercise that Jones dubbed "Proper Strength Training." Cadets were pushed to momentary muscle failure at every station and then rushed to the next. They spit and spewed and turned colors the Academy had never seen. *"For all practical purposes,"* claimed Peterson, *"the intensity of the workouts was so severe that it would have been impossible to appreciably extend them. During the first workouts a few of the subjects became nauseated, but after several weeks of training, not only had such negative reactions entirely disappeared, but the average time to complete a comparable workout had been considerably shortened."* Colonel Al Rushatz, second in command in the Department of Physical Education, joined in the training and commented after the fact, *"I had never worked so hard, nor seen anyone worked to the level the cadets achieved."*

The results of the study astounded the scientists who conducted the testing. After six weeks of training, the Nautilus-Only group increased the resistance used in their exercises (same number of repetitions and exercise sequence as the initial workout) by a minimum of 45% and maximum of 70%—for an average of 58.54%. This more than doubled the results of strength studies conducted during the 1960's and 70's and prompted a comment by Jones: *"If I ever produced only a 25% gain in strength from a 12-week program (as with the average study), I would probably go insane and kill all of the subjects."* At the same time, cadets in the Nautilus-Only group decreased their training time per session by between 4.5-9 minutes, with the average workout lasting just less than thirty minutes.

Strength training is often ignored by coaches and athletes because it is falsely linked to flexibility loss. In this study, proper strength training resulted in flexibility gains that were ten to twenty times that of the Control group on three measures: trunk flexion, trunk extension and shoulder flexion. The average increase with the Nautilus-Only group was 11%; the Control group, .85%.

Cardiovascular fitness was measured under three conditions: *at rest* (heart rate, systolic and diastolic blood pressures, and systolic tension time index [STTI]—a measure of coronary circulation), *during sub-maximal work* (using a bicycle ergometer and a continuous EKG reading, similar to a stress test) and *during maximal work* (total riding time on a bike and the two-mile-run times). All measurements were taken without any knowledge of who was in what group. On **every** test (of sixty), the Nautilus-Only group was superior to the Control group by no small margin. When a summary of the results was plunked on Dr. Cooper's desk, he called them "impossible" and threw them in the trash can. At the time Cooper believed strength training had little to no cardiovascular value. When Jones got word of the discard, he called. The conversation may have been the only thing more brutal than the training, along these lines and minus the expletives: *"The results are impossible, Dr. Cooper, the stupid way you do things. They are only possible by Proper Strength Training."* Captain Peterson backed Jones in his summary: *"The* *data suggests that some of these cardiovascular benefits apparently cannot be achieved by any other type of training."*

With regard to body composition, the Nautilus-Only cadets lost more body fat than those in the Control group.

The results of Project Total Conditioning (detailed in the ATHLETIC JOURNAL, Vol. 56 September, 1975), were spectacular, but were they functional? Did they "work?" Apart from the scientific evaluations, three performance tests were administered: ONE, a two-mile run on the track favored the Nautilus-Only group who improved more than four times (4.32 X) that of the Control group, lowering their time by eighty-eight seconds, compared to twenty; TWO, on a forty-yard dash, the Nautilus-Only group prevailed by improving nearly twice (1.89 X) that of the Control group; THREE, a vertical-jump test revealed that the Nautilus-Only group was more than four times (4.57 X) better than the Control group. Aren't "running faster" and "jumping higher" current goals of functional and sport-specific programs?

How "functional" was the cardiovascular result? The Nautilus-Only group demonstrated lower heart rates at *all* sub-maximal levels (which indicated greater efficiency), a greater work output before heart rates reached 170 beats per minute and longer total bike-ride times (better endurance and less stress at maximal levels). Essentially, they performed at more efficient effort-levels and lasted longer than their counterparts. Isn't that functional?

"The study made it clear," concluded Captain Peterson, *"that high-intensity (weight) training is the most efficient conditioning method known that simultaneously develops high degrees of aerobic and anaerobic conditioning. It offers increases in size and strength, as well as cardiovascular improvement."*

Mike Mentzer (Mr. Universe, 1978) concurred. *"In the past I've alleged that the field of exercise science is a sham, with some of the most celebrated studies never having taken place. Since Project Total Conditioning in 1975, after millions more dollars were spent to develop the most precise testing devices possible—more than 60 other research projects have been conducted, all of which proved essentially the same thing: the overwhelming superiority of brief, high-intensity resistance training for enhancing total fitness. In addition, while most of the studies have been published in scientific journals, the results continue to be ignored, for the most part, by aerobic advocates because they contradict what they've been espousing for decades."* [2]

Many likened the concept of developing high levels of steady-state (aerobic) conditioning from non steady-state (strength) exercise to killing two birds with one stone. They were wrong. It killed a third bird Jones called "metabolic conditioning," the direct cause of that line of bodies strewn across the floor in Lake Helen. It was a higher order of conditioning that no one apparently had—*"the ability to work at 100% intensity for a prolonged time."* And while Jones believed that his tools were superior to what had gone before, he understood that the concept was not exclusive to the use of Nautilus machines.

In his 1978 book, *Conditioning for Football*, Ellington Darden described a method to obtain metabolic conditioning using high-school equipment and three powerful exercise choices: sprints, chin-ups and dips. His plan involved placing numerous chin-up stations (with steps to assist) at one end of the field and dip stations (with similar steps) at the other. Athletes would sprint 100 yards and perform a set of chin-ups (by number or by time), immediately sprint back to perform a set of dips at the other end of the field and continue. The ultimate goal was to perform twelve sprints (of fifteen to twenty seconds) and six sets each of chin-ups and dips (forty to forty-five seconds)—for a total of approximately twelve minutes. If athletes could not perform eight chin-ups or dips, they would do a negative version of the same using the steps. The grueling routine came with a warning: Athletes should be ready (in decent condition) before they start. The efficiency of the plan would eliminate the perceived need of conditioning drills common to the sport. Can you imagine the edge a football team would have with that degree of physical conditioning? They could run a no huddle, non-stop offense that would have their opponents resemble corporal behavior in Lake Helen. Has anyone tried it? And if not, why? The answer is simple: Its application is non-traditional.

Despite the statistical success of its outcome, Project Total Conditioning attracted limited interest. Machine training was new—and "new" to football. The concepts of "high-intensity," "muscle failure" and "brief" were also new.

And if you think minor skill change is difficult, try changing the traditions of a sport or of an industry. The coaching community had a better way, just as "functional" advocates believe they have a better way.

I'll guarantee one thing: If a similar study was conducted today (to borrow the words of Captain Peterson) *"to examine the elative effectiveness of different methods of strength training; and (more importantly) to identify the consequences of a functional training program,"* it wouldn't be close. The potential for increased strength, flexibility, injury-protection and body-composition results through functional training would be pitiful with a capital "P" and worse than traditional studies *before* Project Total Conditioning. The best result (if not the only one) that can be produced by functional training—increased cardiovascular ability—would pale in comparison to that produced in the West-Point study. Only one factor would equate: The skill gained by functional training would equal that gained by Proper Strength Training—NONE. And how would they measure results? By asking if their golf has improved? By re-assessing their ability to perform an overhead squat which would ONLY demonstrate improvement in the performance of an overhead squat? Idiots.

Jones once said, *"If you want to discover how something works, don't focus on what you can do with it. Focus on what you can't do without it."* There is nothing you can't do *without* functional training.

Athletes *don't* need something better—and there is nothing in any case: **Strengthen the muscles you use in your sport, and then practice your sport.**

It's simple and "works" better than anything before or since.

> **"If you want to discover how something works, don't focus on what you can do with it. Focus on what you can't do without it." There is nothing you can't do *without* functional training.**

REFERENCES

[1]   Peterson, J.A., Ph.D., "Total Conditioning: A Case Study," *Athletic Journal*, Vol. 56 September, 1975.

[2]   Mentzer, M., "Aerobics: Myths, Lies and Misconceptions," *Heavy Duty*, 1993.

CHAPTER 15

Sport-Specific Training

Strength is general, and contributes to any activity . . . but the applied demonstration of strength is specific; and learning to apply your strength properly in any activity requires skill training . . . not strength training, but skill training can come from only one possible source, the practice of the sport itself.

Arthur Jones

T he grade-school dropout at the podium was adverse to neckties and protocol: *"We're all ignorant because there are many concepts we are not familiar with,"* he began. *"If I'm in possession of some valuable information you don't have, then I'm at fault if I don't make it available to you. But once I explain the material in a clear, logical manner, then the new pathway should be self-evident to an elementary school student or even a chimpanzee."*

The audience, a mix of staff and students at Duke University, had never heard such an introduction.

"On the other hand," he continued, *"if, after you've heard the facts and had time to reflect, you've chosen to ignore or reject them, that's your fault. Now, you are no longer ignorant. You're stupid. And stupidity goes clear to the bone!"*

Nautilus inventor Arthur Jones could tolerate the former (ignorance), but not the latter. *"Stupidity,"* he added, *"just might get you a personal escort—by me—to the back alley for a good ass-kicking."*

According to Ellington Darden, Ph.D., a member of Jones' entourage that day that included Dick Butkus (NFL Hall of Fame) and Casey Viator (Mr. America, 1971), *"Attendees didn't know whether to laugh or walk out."* Things got worse.

Jones spewed facts and figures, intimidating the crowd as only he could. He insulted those in front because they were close, embarrassed those in back for not sitting up front and harassed those in the middle for being (as Darden suggested) *". . . in the middle."*

Following a three-hour barrage, the history professor who organized the event (and whose protocol was ignored) stood up and suggested a lunch break. The motion was at once interrupted by a student who could not stay for the afternoon and requested his say "now." Jones agreed and listened as the long-haired Ph.D. candidate in physics began to critique his high-intensity training theories.

One minute in, Arthur interrupted, *"I like to do only two things, young man: lecture and fist-fight. Did you want to do the latter before or after lunch?"*

The audience reacted with catcalls; the grad student disappeared.

Jones despised political correctness and loved the value of shock. His approach often "grabbed your attention" whether you agreed with him or not. It grabbed mine . . . and I wasn't alone.

Michael Fulton, M.D., orthopedic representative for Jones' commercial entities, first met Arthur in 1972 and disagreed with him on a range of topics—from physiological concepts at the cellular level to training application at the practical end. Years later Fulton confessed that *in every case* Arthur eventually proved himself right—by logic, by creating tools that measured elusive physiological parameters, by relentless experimentation and inquiry, by stirring things in a fertile mind and, finally, by sharing the "valuable information" with the world.

The article that first caught my attention was "Specificity in Strength Training . . . The Facts and Fables." (*Athletic Journal*, May, 1977). Jones hit hard and fast.

"Don't be misled . . . and you might be on the subject of specificity.

There are no degrees to specificity . . . either you have it or you don't. A movement is utterly specific, or it isn't specific at all.

This being true, as it is, it obviously follows that the only possible way to produce specificity in anything is by performing the act itself. In effect, the only possible specific training for basketball is the act of playing basketball . . . the only possible specific training for swimming is swimming itself, and so on.

Strength is general, and contributes to any activity . . . but the applied demonstration of strength is specific; and learning to apply your strength properly in any activity requires skill training. Which skill training can come from only one possible source, the practice of the sport itself."

And later . . . *"An exercise that is NEARLY specific will simply mess up your skills . . . an exercise that is ALMOST specific will have the same bad result. So don't try to be specific in your exercises . . . doing so is impossible in any case, and the closer you come the greater the danger of hurting your skill.*

Build strength in the best way possible . . . with little or absolutely no regard to how that strength is to be used; then learn to use that strength to your greatest advantage in the only way possible, by practice of the sport itself."

". . . Specificity in strength training is an outright myth, an utter impossibility . . . and it's a good thing that it is impossible, because it has absolutely no value in the way of increasing strength; and . . . anything approaching specificity is even worse, because it will do little or nothing to increase strength but it will hurt your skills.

Some of the same people who are doing so much talking recently about the supposed advantages of specificity in strength training are also responsible for the spreading of other fables of equal value . . . that is to say, no value."

The following chart provides a summary of the fundamental differences between strength and skill training as discussed in Chapter 12:

	STRENGTH TRAINING	SKILL TRAINING
OVERLOAD	Maximum	Zero
INTENSITY	Maximum	Low to Moderate
SPECIFICITY	No	Yes
DURATION/FREQUENCY	Brief, Infrequent	Brief, Frequent

Despite these basic differences, current trends in exercise go a long way to verify another comment by Jones, *"The only thing we learn from history is that we don't learn from history"* (with apologies to Duke's professor). Forty years have passed and "specificity" is common to many strength regimens.

Specificity

In the late 1950's the discipline of "Motor Learning" (how we learn skills) established that motor abilities and skills are specific to a task and that being good at one task does not make one good at another. Moreover, it established that when skills change, the underlying abilities that support the skills must change to meet the new demands.

When many muscles are involved in a skill, the force contribution of each must remain proportionate to the others to retain movement control. As greater resistance is applied to an established skill, the force within each muscle must increase to preserve the proportion, and ultimately, the quality of movement. If the change in resistance (or velocity) alters the motor program—the mechanics—the proportion of force within each muscle must change to accommodate movement efficacy in what has now become a "new" motor program.

Rushall and Pyke affirm its application, *"The principle of specificity states that the maximum benefits of a training stimulus can only be obtained when it replicates the movements and energy systems involved in the activities of a* sport. This principle may suggest that there is no better training than actually performing in the sport" [1]

As true as it is, the notion does not sit well with everyone. *"That abilities are very specific, and that skills do not correlate with each other unless they are virtually identical,"* claims professor, Richard A. Schmidt, Ph.D., *"are often troublesome to students because they do not, at first glance, appear to agree with a number of common observations."* [2]

One such observation—that exercise can enhance athleticism. To be clear: ONLY THE GENERAL NATURE OF EXERCISE (an increase in muscle mass and strength)—NOT ITS SKILL-BASED COMPONENTS—CONTRIBUTES TO GREATER FUNCTION.

Why, then, do so many trainers and athletes mix the two—when the skill component makes NO contribution to improved performance and dilutes the only productive factor, the strength gained through exercise? The answer among sport-specific gurus is clear: "Traditional training is *not enough.*" Then they tour the country converting disciples to bobble-head dolls.

Machines are evil, they say, by subjecting muscles to an "artificial" environment, to isolation, to a single-movement track, to balanced resistance and they don't allow feet to touch the floor. The list goes on. The "experts" prefer pulleys, bands and free-weights to replicate skill patterns through a variety of movement planes—unaware of the consequences.

Tim Wakeham, Assistant Strength and Conditioning Coach of the Michigan State Spartans, explains:

"Since movements with resistance added to them are no longer replications, does it matter what resistance mode is used for enhancing sport performances? Everything is non-functional when it comes to producing a meaningful (skill) transfer.

According to my reading, transfer appears to drop dramatically when even one factor between the training mode and performance differs. Everything from free weights, machines, medicine balls and resistance bands, share many differences when compared to actual sport performance.

Some coaches have professed that free weights have a greater ability to produce statistically significant transfer to performance when compared to machines.

I'd be interested in reading the definitive, unbiased, valid and reliable research. If a free-weight exercise does transfer more than its machine counterpart, how much more transfer are we talking about? If the free-weight exercise transfers 10% of usable adaptation while the machine transfers 6%, is this a meaningful difference?" [3] No such research exists.

Jones hit the nail on the head, *"There are no degrees to specificity . . . either you have it or you don't. A movement is utterly specific, or it isn't specific at all."* Despite the clarity, many find it difficult to distinguish specific from non-specific, struggle to accept the nonexistence of transfer or simply believe otherwise. If trainers, coaches and athletes ever get their collective heads out of the sand, they will quickly discover that they don't have far to look for answers.

Specificity and Motor Learning: "Practice Makes Perfect"

"Practice makes perfect, but only if you practice perfectly," affirms a Motor-Learning staple—the SAID Principle (Specific Adaptation to Imposed Demand)—that specificity of learning lends itself to specificity of practice. To become good at something requires specific learning; to become better requires more specific practice. If you practice the squat but rarely the lunge or hack squat, for example, the greatest gains in ability and lifting proficiency occur with the squat. Performance in the lunge and hack-squat may increase when tested, but progress is likely the result of an overall increase in lean muscle tissue (strength) from the squat—and has little to do with the assumed transfer of proficiency in squats to other exercises. An increase in muscle strength means an increase in function that transfers to activities (exercises) apart from those routinely practiced. Conversely,

> **Build strength in the best way possible . . . with little or absolutely no regard to how that strength is to be used; then learn to use that strength to your greatest advantage in the only way possible, by practice of the sport itself.**

a surge in performance due to an increase in neurological function (skill, without lean muscle gain) results in greater lifting proficiency in the exercises practiced but less strength transfer to other exercises.

The "assumption" of *skill crossover* or *transfer* from one activity to another violates the SAID principle. Stronger muscles can improve performance. Yet, many believe that strengthening muscles as they move in the same motion as their sport (or activity of choice) can *better* improve performance. Not so. If a person performs an exercise that is *similar* in nature—but not performed *exactly* as in the activity the person wants to improve—there is NO crossover, NO transfer. Changing the conditions under which a task is performed enables a person to get better at a "new"—but not the original—task.

Arthur Jones explains:

"Adding a few ounces to the weight of a basketball will do absolutely nothing in the way of increasing your strength for playing basketball . . . but it will certainly mess up your skill at basketball. Adding a few pounds to the weight of a basketball will do very little in the way of increasing your strength . . . and it will still have some bad effect on your skill, although not as much as the previous example.

So it is obvious that the closer we come to having specificity (in exercise), the worse off we are . . . until and unless we have total specificity, in which case we are simply throwing a normal basketball in our usual fashion; which will increase our skill while doing nothing for our strength." [4]

The sport of football is particularly liable to matching exercises with movements on the field. To be clear: Other than the strength gained by either, there is no correlation between a single exercise and a single sporting activity. Is the "power clean" (mentioned in Chapter 11) more effective for strength and development in football than other exercises? Probably not. Is the risk of injury greater with the power clean than other exercises? Probably so. And if so, it's only value is personal preference.

> **. . . there is no correlation between a single exercise and a single sporting activity.**

The intricacies (what is correct) and deviations (what can go wrong) of each skill pattern are specific. Resistance added to a skill makes the pattern non-specific and non-specific activity, *even if it appears similar*, CANNOT contribute to the skill(s) of another activity. For best results from both, strength training and skill training MUST remain apart.

Specificity and Muscle Soreness

A marathon runner in Caracas mounted a Nordic Track® cross-country ski machine in my gym and lasted five minutes. Likewise dozens of Venezuelan bodybuilders tried Nautilus machines for the first time with the same results. In both cases, difference of movement—not superiority of equipment—led to their demise. The "new" movements were non-specific and resulted in what Rushall and Pyke described as: *"Muscle soreness in recovery; acute localized fatigue during the activity; a rapid occurrence of fatigue; and a subjective appraisal that the work was harder than usual."* [5]

Tim Wakeham theorized the same with the Michigan State football team. *"If I started training athletes using functional movements (that mimic sport-movement patterns) at the midpoint of their season, every athlete would feel soreness."* Why? The mimicking exercises are different, NON-SPECIFIC. If they were specific (exactly the same), the muscles would NOT be unusually sore.

This, in part, explains the attraction of non-traditional exercise in gyms—Pilates, Yoga, TRX, Zumba or whatever the latest. First-time exposure to non-specific exercise creates muscle soreness which many hail a plus—a natural mistake. Non-specific is *different* and different can create soreness without a positive effect on performance.

A Specific Conclusion

For the most part, the literature on motor learning shows that the greatest increases between training and performance occur when variables are held constant—same exercises, types of exercise (isometric, concentric, etc.), ranges of motion and movement velocity (to a lesser degree).

Hence, the best way to increase performance (reaction time, power, agility, balance or coordination in any sport or activity) is to practice skills specifically as one intends to demonstrate those skills. Greater function (to better demonstrate proficiency, not skill) can be obtained through general weight-training. In effect, an increase in lean muscle mass from machine or free-weight use within stable environments lends itself to better demonstrate ability outside the weight room than functional training or sport-specific exercises. However, the specificity of weight-training movements is irrelevant to the skills demonstrated in tasks outside of weight training. The exception is the practice of lifting weights for the sport of power-lifting (the practice of specific resistance training skills for competition).

Speed of Movement

Another "fable" Jones exposed in his article on specificity was speed of movement during exercise. *"How fast one moves while performing exercises for the purpose of building strength,"* he said, *"has absolutely nothing to do with how fast one can move while using the strength of those same muscles."*

Others disagree. *"Specificity of training,"* claims Donald A. Chu, spokesperson for the NSCA (National Strength and Conditioning Association, a trainer "certification" group), *"tells us that if you train slowly, you move slowly, and if you desire to increase speed of movement you had better include speed training in your program"*—the NSCA interpretation of the SAID Principle.

Jones called it his way, *"Hogwash, pure unadulterated garbage, utterly false and dangerously misleading misinformation."*

Who's right? You decide. Add weight to an exercise and speed of movement decreases: Nothing else is possible. You can lift ten pounds quickly, 100 pounds less quickly and your car, not quickly at all. Yet, Chu and others claim that speed of movement in a task increases by practicing at a speed that is slower than possible due to the resistance added during exercise. Baseball pitchers, for example, routinely perform explosive chest (or shoulder) presses with a light-to-moderate resistance to increase throwing velocity. If the resistance weighs more than a baseball (and it generally does), the process only serves to *decrease* speed of movement compared to that of throwing a baseball.

Using that logic, explosive weight-lifting should make an athlete SLOWER, not faster, since most sports activities consist of limb speeds that are faster than those possible during exercise. Yet, Chu insists: *"To deny the effects of plyometric (explosive) training is to deny the obvious."*

The "obvious" is this, Mr. Chu: Strength gains are minimized by "explosive" speeds of movement during exercise (in essence, resistance must be lifted—not thrown—to stimulate change); "fast" exposes muscle/joint system(s) to high forces; and, the ONLY direct result of "explosive" training is injury.

And it doesn't end there.

SPORTS-PERFORMANCE PROGRAMS

The popularity of the word "performance" should raise a red flag in the field of exercise. Sports-performance programs stack-up to the largest fraud in the history of exercise—the 1921 "Kick-Sand-In-Your-Face/Dynamic-Tension" training system of Charles Atlas.

Sports-performance programs imply several negatives: ONE, they violate the concept of "specificity" in motor learning by replicating sports movements against resistance which can interfere with the skills involved; TWO, they limit strength gains by restricting the choice of exercise tools to those that allow movement through multiple planes, restrict exercises to multi-joint movements and limit work intensity by their moronic philosophy; THREE, they promote explosive speed of movement during exercise, especially in sports that require the production of "power;" and FOUR, they introduce athletes to the ultimate insanity, impact.

I worked in a MedX-equipped facility in Jupiter, Florida that rented space to a sports-performance group called "Ultimate Speed®." Their directors held Master's degrees in Exercise Science which justified a conclusion Jones often reached, *"There is no education but self-education."* The incessant clang of weights heralded the construction of anything but athletes.

One day, NBA Hall-of-Fame player and coach, Bill Cunningham and I watched as the "experts" attached a high-school athlete to a device designed to increase vertical jump. The "Power Jumper" connected a platform base to the waist of the trainee by a series of latex tubes that allowed vertical leaps against resistance. *"During my playing days,"* Cunningham chuckled, *"we had a salesman drop by to promote a similar device. Coach agreed to give it a try, so we used it several times a week after practice."* To make a long story short, the team's ability to jump was significantly reduced, with Bill losing "several inches."

Rushall and Pyke explain why: *"Adjustments to technique to handle the minor loads (of extra-load training) might produce negative training effects because of the subtle alteration to refined neuromuscular movement patterns. Extra-load resistances used on the extremities have not been shown to be of value for training."* [6]

In plain English, resistance added to movement patterns may screw up your skill.

Another observation: It doesn't require a Master's degree to generate sports-performance ideas. A hockey player walks in and hockey-like exercises appear. Tennis, tennis-like movements; golf, you got it. And parents beam that little Johnny has finally discovered a place to flourish into his athletic best. After all, the staff is qualified and exercises are *just like* hockey, tennis, golf . . .

"Just like" is NOT the way to go.

Research and Observations

Skill and strength training do NOT mix. Examine this conclusion from research on summer training for speed skaters . . . *"neither low walking (a walking-like movement in a skating position) nor dry skating (side-to-side, deep sitting push-offs) can be considered as specific training activities for speed skaters. There are no valuable training effects that will enhance speed skating from the enactment of these activities. They are useless activities for competent skaters. They could even be counter-productive if emphasized too heavily (probably would cause disruption of high-level neuromuscular patterns)." [7]*

And, examine the conclusion of a study on swimmers who trained against additional resistance in the pool: *"Costill, Sharp, and Troup (1980) concluded that swimming strength is best achieved by repeated maximum exercises that duplicate as closely as possible the skill of swimming. The most appropriate exercise that they suggested was a series of maximum sprint swims." [8]*

Another swimming study (1985) examined the effect of resistance on mechanics. They filmed four male and two female groups as they sprinted the butterfly (approximately forty feet) under three conditions: normal, partially resisted (tethered by a swim belt) and sprint-assisted (using a tethered belt). A biomechanical analysis revealed:

1. Sprint-resisted training caused a shorter and slower stroke.
2. Sprint-assisted training increased the stroke rate (shortened stroke length, not hand velocity).
3. Both forms of training changed stroke mechanics and cast doubt on their efficacy.

The study concluded that the resisted and assisted training methods were counter-productive. Each (method) encouraged swimmers to adopt less efficient mechanics. [9]

Ask a football coach about his team's first practice in full or partial uniform. The timing and coordination of plays without pads is suddenly compromised by the weight of what the athletes wear. They are slower; the team is slower. The added resistance disrupts the skill established in shirt sleeves—the "good" news. If you link to a performance program that embraces the production of "power" (and most do), you will find yourself performing not only movements against resistance, but "explosive" movements against resistance—the "bad" news.

One day an Ultimate Speed® director sat a high-school teen on a MedX Avenger® (plate-loaded) chest-press machine with clear instructions, "Explode," then seconds later and louder, "EXPLODE." While that echoed in my left ear, advice from Arthur Jones resonated in my right. *"The next time somebody suggests that you move suddenly during any form of either exercise or testing, smile and walk away, because you are talking to a fool. And do not overlook the fact that a very long list of fools has large muscles, and another long list of fools has all sorts of academic credentials."*

Arthur often measured the degree of foolishness with his force plate/ oscilloscope demonstrations described in Chapter 6. Whether you sat in front or back, the result was always the same: LIFTING WEIGHTS RAPIDLY IS *NOT* PRODUCTIVE AND *NOT* SAFE.

Despite the obvious, many trainers and athletes advocate the use of—and claim to extract the desired training effect from—explosive movements. But that claim may be skewed, as research suggests:

"Grabe and Widule (1988) determined that much of the training effect from explosive power training is due to the motor learning of the skill associated with the activity. The actual activities of the sport would seem to be the best training exercises for the development of both speed and power." [10]

And (from the same source) . . .

"Training for power and speed would seem to be relatively simple. The activity itself should form the basis of the form of movement, the technique should be as economical as possible, and given the restrictions of this, the action should be as intense as possible. Anything less than a maximum effort will train different neuromuscular patterns and should be considered counterproductive." [10]

The next time somebody suggests that you move suddenly during either any form of exercise or testing, smile and walk away, because you are talking to a fool. And do not overlook the fact that a very long list of fools has large muscles, and another long list of fools has all sorts of academic credentials.

Despite clear proof, many sports-performance advocates insist that explosive movements and plyometric activities (jumping on or over boxes from various levels, jump squats, etc.) are safe and productive; and that their programs follow the SAID principle to the letter. Their logic is simple—*to prepare the body for the high forces of impact (in sports), you must expose it to—or practice—impact (such as that encountered during plyometric activities).* My logic is likewise simple. My daily drive to and from work involves travel on a dangerous highway, I-95. The high probability of an accident requires that I prepare for the inevitable by ramming my car into the wall adjacent to the parking lot each day after work. I know one thing: My car won't last long. And another: The body comes with a limited warranty. And a third: Trainers and coaches just don't get it.

Arthur Jones used several analogies to expose the danger of plyometrics and explosive training:

- *"Jump from your bathroom vanity onto your scale to see how much you weigh. In the air you'll weigh nothing; when you land, you might weigh several thousand pounds."*
- *"Plyometrics is the equivalent of running athletes to the top of the stadium stairs and having them jump into the parking lot."*
- *"Anyone dumb enough to do plyometrics will get exactly what they deserve—hurt."*

To add insult to injury, the impact encountered during plyometric activities is *different* from that encountered on a football field. And different means *non-specific*. Exposure to plyometric activity A, for example, results in the body's adaptation to the demands of plyometric activity A. Exposure to plyometric activity B results in adaptation to the demands of plyometric activity B. And, other than the strength gained through the practice of plyometric activities A and B (which is minimal due to the momentum created), plyometrics does NOT prepare the body for the demands of impact encountered on the field. Each football impact is unique—different forces at different angles imposed on different body parts—which makes specific preparation impossible. The only thing that prepares the body for the demands of impact is to increase the integrity of the muscle/joint system(s) to resist force (by strength training). Outside of that, exposure to the impact encountered on the football field prepares the body for the demands encountered on the football field (according to the SAID principle). The assumption of transfer from plyometric activities to sports performance DOES NOT EXIST—which makes many football traditions look as foolish as they are.

Conclusion

On January 27, 2012, The Golf Channel's *Inside the PGA Tour®* featured clips of touring pro, John Mallinger's fitness routine. One clip showed him standing on a balance board while his instructor urged him to find his center, keep his balance and take a full swing with a golf club—*useless, unless John takes the board with him on the course.* Another showed him jumping laterally over a low box or bench—*the same activity that, in 1999, injured the left knee of Mariner shortstop, Alex Rodriguez, also supervised by a "certified" strength coach who believed in plyometrics.* A third showed John juggling tennis balls as he stood on a Bosu Ball—*an audition for the Barnum and Bailey Open, but utterly useless for golf.* Nonsense has no limit . . . an opinion shared by others.

"As a teacher of motor learning, and someone whose Ph.D. is in the area of skill learning," says Dave Smith, a Lecturer in Sport Psychology at Chester College (UK), *"I am increasingly frustrated by the number of strength coaches and others who advocate training methods, such as Swiss-ball training, that violate the most basic motor learning principles, particularly in regards to specificity. It is sad that such scientifically unsound and unproductive methods have gained such prominence, and (incredibly) acceptance in the coaching community. Anyone who advocates such methods clearly has little basic understanding of motor learning, and should not be coaching or providing advice on technical coaching matters."* [11]

Jones said it his way. *"Bullshit is rather easy to establish, and once established, almost impossible to eradicate."*

The formula to increase performance (and *"power"*) in sports is simple:

1. **Increase skill.**
2. **Increase strength in the muscles used.**
3. **Keep strength training *totally independent* of skill training.**
4. **Decrease overall body fat (which acts as friction during muscle contraction).**

Unfortunately, simple doesn't sell.

REFERENCES

[1] Rushall, B.S., Pyke, F.S., *Training for Sports and Fitness*, Melbourne, Australia: Macmillan of Australia, 1991.

[2] Johnston, B.D., System Analysis, Bodyworx Publishing, 177, 2001.

[3] Johnston, B.D., System Analysis, Bodyworx Publishing, 173, 2001.

[4] Jones, A., "Specificity in Strength Training—The Facts and Fables," *Athletic Journal*, May, 1977.

[5] Rushall, B.S., Pyke, F.S., *Training for Sports and Fitness*, Melbourne, Australia: Macmillan of Australia, 1991.

[6] Rushall, B.S., Pyke, F.S., *Training for Sports and Fitness*, Melbourne, Australia: Macmillan of Australia, 1991.

[7] DeBoer, R.W., Ettema, G.J., Faessen, B.G., Krekels, H., Hollander, A.P., De Groot, G., Van Ingen Schenau, G.I., "Specific Characteristics of Speed Skating: Implications for Summer Training." *Medicine and Science in Sports and Exercise*, 19, 504-510, 1987.

[8] Rushall, B.S., Pyke, F.S., *Training for Sports and Fitness*, Melbourne, Australia: Macmillan of Australia, 1991.

⁹ Maglischo, E.W., Maglischo, C.W., Zier, D.J., Santos, T.R., "The Effects of Sprint-Assisted and Sprint-Resisted Swimming on Stroke Mechanics." *Journal of Swimming Research*, 1 27-33, 1985.

¹⁰ Rushall, B.S., Pyke, F.S., *Training for Sports and Fitness*, Melbourne, Australia: Macmillan of Australia, 1991.

¹¹ Johnston, B.D., System Analysis, Bodyworx Publishing, 177, 2001.

CHAPTER 16

···

The Strength/Performance Connection

When I started "lifting weights" in 1962, I purchased six exercise charts from Weider of Canada,® pinned them to the basement wall and pounded away three times a week. Fifteen years later I had not missed a session. As an aspiring athlete I somehow thought it would do me good but failed to realize the degree to which I had plunged into the minority. My friends didn't lift and only a handful of upperclassmen were rumored to be lifting at home. It wasn't popular and—I didn't know at the time—was feared all the way from my high school to the upper echelon of professional sports.

The fear was that big muscles would make athletes incompetent in anything other than "lifting weights." Coaches were convinced it had no value—would *hurt* performance—and were unwilling to gamble. The NFL didn't use barbells until the late 1960's. The introduction of Nautilus machines a few years later made the process more acceptable and the promise of greater results eventually attracted the coaching community. Don Shula's resounding success with the Miami Dolphins in the early 1970's helped pave the way to a general acceptance of "lifting weights" for athletic performance.

But it didn't end the skepticism, as Arthur Jones pointed out:

"As a result of the widespread fear of exercise and a lack of factual information on the subject of exercise, most coaches and athletes are overlooking a very important factor . . . while continuing to labor under the mistaken belief that they are doing everything possible *in the direction*

of improving functional ability. The edge that most coaches are constantly looking for has been in plain sight for a long time . . . but remains largely untapped, unsuspected, even feared, and certainly misunderstood.

. . . sometime In the far distant future, people will look back on the present era of sports as the age of ignorance . . . primarily because of the lack of attention now being given to the intelligent use of exercise. Most athletes still finish their careers with absolutely nothing in the way of strength training . . . and very few (if any) athletes are producing 50% of the potential benefit of a properly conducted program of exercise." [1]

Forty years have passed and things haven't changed. In an attempt to attract people, the fitness industry has all but destroyed the potential benefits of exercise by sweeping strength training under the carpet. They first catered to females who feared big muscles by introducing activities that purport to "sculpt and tone"—the perfect audible for their target. They introduced equipment to skirt the drudgery of lifting weights—Swiss Balls, TRX straps, vibrating platforms, heavy ropes and hundreds of colorful gadgets that require nothing more than bodyweight to produce "great" advertized results. It threw free-weights and machines into an uphill battle to prove their "functional" application. After all, how does sitting on a machine and lifting a weight through a fixed plane help a golf swing that requires feet on the ground and a distinct movement pattern?

The industry has brainwashed the public to believe that traditional training is inferior to other choices, to the point that those choices have become distractions. The process has diluted the strength component and all but destroyed the production of best results from exercise. Strength should be the focus . . . but is not.

Jones believed that functional ability was a product of five factors: Strength, skill, bodily proportions, cardiovascular ability and neurological efficiency—and that strength was the only "productive" factor. Below, he discusses the interrelationship of the five factors and the importance of muscular strength to performance:

"No amount of muscle will help an athlete much if he lacks the skill to use it effectively . . . but no amount of muscle will hurt his skill either; instead,

increasing his strength will always improve his functional ability, in any sport.

An athlete's muscles can be as strong as those of an elephant . . . but if his bodily proportions are bad for a particular sport, then he will still not be able to perform well. But he will, at least perform better than he would have with weaker muscles.

A sprinter can have muscles like those of Hercules and still fall flat on his face after a 100-yard dash if his cardiovascular condition is bad . . . but he should not make the common mistake of assuming that he can have only one or the other, either great strength or good cardiovascular condition but not both. In fact, it is easily possible and highly desirable to have both.

One of the most outstanding muscular freaks that I ever saw was actually a fairly weak man . . . stronger than an average man, but certainly not as strong as one might guess from the size of his muscles. But his lack of strength is in no way related to the size of his muscles; as it happens, this particular individual is very low on the scale of neurological ability; he lacks the ability to utilize a large part of his actual muscle mass . . . a genetic problem that is not subject to improvement.

But even this man, weak as he is, is still far more capable than he would have been with smaller, weaker muscles.

. . . In the meantime, it has been clearly and repeatedly demonstrated hundreds of times, with no single exception I ever heard of and no exception I would believe unless I saw it myself, that proper strength training will markedly improve the performance of any athlete in any sport.

And the great athletes are the ones who have the most to gain from strength training . . . and are the most unlikely to use it; having been falsely convinced that it will hurt them. Proper strength training may improve the functional ability of a clod by as much as 50 percent . . . but he will still be a clod, and will still be run over by untrained athletes who have all of the natural advantages that the clod lacks. But even a 2 percent improvement in the functional ability of a natural athlete may well be the difference between a good athlete and a world champion." [2]

I first learned about functional ability as a sixteen-year-old junior golfer when I was paired with a reputable peer in Toronto. Ken Trowbridge, a Dan Marino lookalike, was my height and weighed about 120 pounds. I'd been lifting weights for two years and was in the process of creating a name for myself. The girth of his arms and wrists was half that of mine—but it was no contest. Ken outdrove me by sixty yards at every tee. I had the strength; he had the skill to generate club-head speed. I've often wondered what I could have accomplished with his skill or what he could have accomplished with my strength.

Two of the five factors that affect functional ability—bodily proportions and neurological efficiency—are not subject to change through training, but the other three are. Let's examine the relationship of strength to skill and cardiovascular ability, things we can change.

An increase in strength through progressive resistance exercise indirectly enhances skill by connecting the nervous system to better tools. As Jones suggests, strength will *always improve* functional ability.

At the same time, an increase in strength triggers a proportionate increase in local muscular endurance—the ability of a muscle to repeat a task. If the task is prolonged to activate a steady-state response, muscle strength becomes a determining factor in cardiovascular training. It may, in fact, be the *limiting* factor in our ability to absorb, transport and utilize oxygen, as described:

"Our ultimate cardiovascular capacity (as our potential for strength) is determined by genetics. A review of oxygen pathways—from absorption in the lungs and transportation through the circulatory system, to consumption by the muscle—can help determine what limits that capacity.

... In the meantime, it has been clearly and repeatedly demonstrated hundreds of times, with no single exception I ever heard of and no exception I would believe unless I saw it myself, that proper strength training will markedly improve the performance of any athlete in any sport.

The purpose of the lungs is to saturate blood with oxygen, a function easily met under all conditions. At rest, total saturation is accomplished in the first third of the blood's transit time through the lung's capillaries. During maximal exercise, with the heart rate and blood flow increased dramatically and transit time reduced by 50%, the reserve capacity of the lungs can easily meet the demand. At the receiving end, muscles are capable of consuming all of the oxygen in the brief period of time it takes the blood to flow through its capillaries, both at rest and during heavy exercise. Therefore, with the lungs and muscles loading and unloading oxygen at near 100% efficiency, neither appears to be a limiting factor.

The same, however, cannot be said of the circulatory system. Many physiologists believe that the heart itself is the limiting factor, reasoning that if the heart could pump more blood, the body would consume more oxygen. Accordingly, the role of cardiovascular exercise should be to increase the effectiveness of the heart's ability to pump blood. Others claim that the heart can only pump the amount of blood returning to it, and that the peripheral blood vessels restrict the blood's return by resisting every attempt the heart makes to increase blood flow.

When a muscle contracts, internal pressure rises and compresses the blood vessels within, restricting flow. Research demonstrates that such restriction begins with a voluntary contraction of as little as 20% and increases proportionately with the intensity of effort. At 50-60% (of a maximum contraction), no blood flow is present—and no oxygen delivered or consumed. The system shuts down.

There are only two ways to decrease muscle-contraction intensity during activity:

- Increase the skill of the individual performing the movement, thereby diminishing the quantity of unnecessary contraction.
- Increase the strength of the muscles involved so that each contraction requires a smaller percentage of the available muscle mass.

Skill is highly specific and requires time to develop, while strength is universal and acquired more efficiently. A distance runner could become a distance swimmer by learning efficient swimming technique. He could improve at both by becoming stronger.

Therefore, in the same way genetic factors dictate our ultimate level of strength, so muscle strength limits our ultimate cardiovascular capacity. Proper strength training should be the focus of every program designed to increase physiological function." [3]

Strength is the cornerstone of every trainable component of functional ability, yet it is rarely given the respect it deserves.

Years ago I worked in an exercise facility in Wellington, Florida, winter home to the horse industry. One day the coach of a prominent Polo Team from Argentina brought his players in for a workout (a twice-weekly event). I was curious. He assembled the men in a circle and led them through a series of grade-school calisthenics that I thought was a warm-up. Wrong. The coach wouldn't let them near the exercise equipment. Professional athletes? Training for polo? Pathetic—but no worse than what I see today.

Most trainees select activities that Jones would call "supportive in nature"—the imaginary skill training inherent in functional exercise; the flexibility orientation of Yoga, Pilates and stretch classes; or the cardiovascular choice of treadmills, elliptical trainers and bikes—all of which have little-to-no strength component. And I can't count the number of clients who have swapped progressive resistance exercise for "one of the above" or "something new," only to return with claims of "lost strength."

One day I stood at the front desk of a fitness center when an elderly gentleman entered and hammered his fist to the counter, "I want to lift some weights." After a few sessions I asked the ninety-three year-old, "What motivated you to come in as you did?" "Well," he said, "a friend of mine passed away a couple of months ago. At the funeral I looked down and said, 'Jimmy, I'm not going to let that happen to me.' He let his mobility down and ended up in bed, then the hospital and gone. It was quick. I want to keep my legs strong so it doesn't happen to me." I was inspired.

With an older population, the focus on balance, flexibility, skill and agility are all "supportive in nature" to what really counts, strength. When muscle strength declines, mobility fades. Soon, you can't get around, can't get up from a chair, from bed—and gone. The cause may be listed as "natural" or "a heart attack," but was really a result of the largest *indirect* cause of death—lack of mobility.

Proper strength training is the step that needs to be taken.

> **You cannot access muscles in a meaningful way via the heart, but you can access the heart in a meaningful way through the muscles.**

REFERENCES

[1] Jones, A., "Improving Functional Ability in any Sport," Peterson, J.A., Ph.D. (editor), *Total Fitness the Nautilus Way*, Leisure Press, 8: 86-88, 1978.

[2] Jones, A., "The Relationship of Strength to Functional Ability in Sports," Peterson, J.A., Ph.D. (editor), *Total Fitness the Nautilus Way*, Leisure Press, 16: 163-166, 1978.

[3] Bannister, G., "The Limits of Cardiovascular Endurance," *In Arthur's Shadow*, Cork Hill Press, Jan. 14: 73, 2005.

CHAPTER 17

···

Core Exercise

Background

I n 1980 I purchased twelve exercise machines to establish the first commercial Nautilus facility in South America. At the time, no machines for the abdomen or lumbar spine were available.

Three years later I visited Nautilus headquarters to purchase thirteen more, including the *new* abdominal and lower-back machines. Their inventor, Arthur Jones, was slow to introduce an "ab" machine because he firmly believed, "the abdomen takes care of itself." (*He built it more as a challenge than a need to "complete" his line*). The lower-back machine was different. At the time it represented eleven years of research and development and was the *first* device to address the important muscles of the lumbar spine. During my visit I was escorted to the showcase gym by a man I later discovered was "Foots" Lee, former center of the Tampa Bay Bucs. I inquired about the abdominal machine. His reply was swift, *"You don't need it. Come with me. I'll run you through eleven machines and put you on it at the end. If you do three repetitions, I'll give you a hundred bucks. That's how hard you'll work your stomach as we go."* It could have been a million—I wasn't about to press my luck.

Around that time Jones developed a computerized version of his lower-back machine that measured strength. The orthopedic representative for Nautilus Sports/Medical Industries, Dr. Michael Fulton, was invited (among others) to present the data gleaned from his research on the device to a special Senate committee in Washington. *Was there a connection between muscle strength and pain perception in the treatment of chronic back pain? Was there a cure for "the most expensive non-life-threatening problem in the field of medicine?"* The answers were the same as the one I recently received by E-mail from a Canadian friend: How many Toronto Maple-Leafs does it take to win the Stanley Cup? *"We don't know and we may never know."* Fulton's presentation fell on deaf ears. The committee was engrossed in the wisdom of invitee Linda Evans, who had just written a new book on exercise—which further confirmed, *"We don't know and we may never know."*

While this was unfolding, I was face-up in a hospital in Caracas, Venezuela, recovering from a second back operation. My long history of issues encountered a longer list of physicians who shared the wisdom, *"Strengthen your abdominals."* So I did. One set, three times a week for four years . . . the same on the lower-back machine. It kept me upright but Jones had something up his sleeve.

My next visit to Florida took me to his new venue, Ocala. Arthur sold Nautilus in 1986 and established a new corporation, MedX, which (originally) produced machines for specific testing and rehabilitative exercise of the knee, lumbar and cervical spines. To market his products, Jones flew medical doctors to his home seven days a week and lectured to them for eight to ten hours to verify his assumption, *"They know nothing."* I attended one lecture, was fascinated by the message and messenger, and stayed for seven. Jones loved truth more than shock—and he loved shock—but his message was clear: *"My (Nautilus) back machine doesn't work,"* and *"Abdominal strength has nothing to do with back pain."* He then backed his statements with data.

On the first point Jones discovered that the majority of subjects who had used his Nautilus Lower-back machine for years in a progressive manner remained in a state of atrophy. The "why" was clear: The Nautilus machine allowed the pelvis to rotate and the large muscles of the hip to activate, which is where the benefit remained. His latest tool—the MedX Lumbar Extension machine—prevented pelvic rotation and directed the stimulus to the small muscles that extend the spine.

Abdominal strength has nothing to do with back pain.

On the second point Jones bucked convention. Twenty years before, electromyography (EMG) studies compared the strength of the lumbar muscles to those of the abdomen and revealed a discrepancy in favor of the lower back. Ever since, the medical community has hung its hat on the belief that the imbalance was related to the high incidence of low-back problems. Jones disagreed. He measured the isolated strength of the muscles that extend the spine in a large and varied population and found nothing but atrophy. The weakness lay with the muscles that extend the spine and subsequent research at the University of Florida demonstrated that the majority of people exposed to valid, *isolated* exercise for the lumbar muscles responded in dramatic fashion—which verified his contention.

The decade before, Jones worked with professional bodybuilders and refused to train abdominals. In 1971 he prepared Casey Viator for the Mr. America contest. Viator won every category but best abdominals despite the fact that his abdominal muscles (confirmed by photos) were on par with any bodybuilder, living or dead. For eleven months before the contest Casey performed ZERO abdominal exercise while his competitors performed millions of repetitions. Jones remained steadfast.

When I returned home I removed both machines from my program and felt no difference. Arthur was on to something.

In 1988 I purchased the MedX Lumbar Extension machine and took it to Caracas, serious about "fixing" my back which had suffered two major crises since the second operation. The last crisis left me with a condition known as "drop foot." After six months of therapy, I was still dragging a foot around. I used the MedX machine as per protocol and in twenty weeks became pain free—and have remained so for twenty-four years. The last 23½ of those years I have used the lumbar frequency suggested by research—once a month for ninety seconds—and the abdominal frequency suggested by Jones, NONE.

Infrequent exercise for the back and none for the front: Just what the doctor(s) ordered.

The Core

Core training probably arrived the same way as functional training: Someone woke up one morning and declared "the core" important—for sports, for everyday activities, for posture, for aesthetics and last but not least, for money. It was suddenly the missing piece of the puzzle. Where did it come from and what research backed it? The birth of core training seemed eerily similar to Paul Chek's description of what occurs as you exercise on his magical Swiss ball: Things *"just happen."*

Someone defined the magic: *"The balanced development of the superficial muscles that stabilize, align and move the trunk of the body, especially the abdominals and muscles of the back."* Core advocates believe, as the medical community before, that spinal muscles are stronger than abdominal muscles, despite a decade of research at the University of Florida that clearly demonstrates the opposite.

"Balanced development" is important for joint stability, but what does it mean and how can it be measured? Would you know *if* and *when* you were balanced? MedX research has established an optimal (normal) strength curve for the isolated muscles that extend the lumbar spine through a full range of motion but the same has never been established for isolated abdominal muscles. *The only valid comparison between isolated, antagonistic muscle groups was published by Arthur Jones in 1993—a comparison of ideal strength curves for front and rear thigh muscles.* [1] Judging from that work, balanced development in the midsection might mean abdominal muscles that are stronger than lumbar muscles at some angles and weaker at others. And the relationship would require frequent measurement to see if you were "balanced," still "balanced" or approaching a "balanced" state.

Without proper tools, the only option is to strengthen muscles to their maximum on all sides of a joint with a device that changes the resistance according to the ideal strength curve of each muscle through a complete range of motion. And that means use of a machine with a proper cam or lever system—which to most is heresy. Core "experts" prefer exercises that *cannot* produce full-range strength OR prefer isometric "holds" that limit strength gain to a few angles. Then they judge their work as follows: If you "feel" better, you just *might* be "balanced."

Judging from the poor strength levels of the majority of low backs tested, it would be hard to imagine that abdominal muscles are in worse condition, which means:

- Those who begin core training have an imbalance to start—an abdomen stronger than low back.
- Because it is impossible to strengthen low-back muscles through traditional means, any attempt to strengthen both sides of the core (front and back) results in the strengthening of abdominals only, which makes the imbalance worse.

Low-Back Muscles

If you buy into core training, as many have, there are problems with *"especially the muscles of the back."* The most important third of the core—the lumbar spine—CANNOT be strengthened in a meaningful way using traditional means. Why? Traditional exercise allows the pelvis to rotate, thereby strengthening hip muscles. The only device that can isolate and meaningfully access the muscles that extend the lumbar spine from a strength perspective is the MedX Lumbar Extension machine. If you don't believe that—and most trainers don't—look up the decade of research from The Center for Exercise Science, University of Florida (1988-1998), then add these stories:

- Jones' new back device represented fourteen years of research, 3,000 prototypes, $88 million and was nominated for a Nobel Prize in medicine. In other words, Arthur didn't wake up one morning and declare it a hit. Dr. Fulton, who was present from day one, provided his medical advice along the way and wrote the following:

  "During the last four years, carefully conducted and large-scale research has clearly proven that less than two minutes of weekly exercise is all that is required in order to strengthen these muscles to a degree that I would not have believed possible as recently as four years ago. Working with this new equipment, using five of our research staff as our first subjects in order to learn what to

expect from later and much-larger-scale research, the results were as follows:

SUBJECT ONE, an increase in the strength of the fully-extended lumbar extension muscles of 180 percent as a result of ten exercises performed over a period of ten weeks. One brief exercise each week.

SUBJECT TWO, an increase of 450 percent as a result of one exercise every fourteen days for a period of five months.

SUBJECT THREE, an increase of 877 percent as a result of one exercise performed approximately every fourteen days for a period of twenty-seven weeks.

SUBJECT FOUR, an increase of 1,460 percent as a result of one exercise every fourteen days for a period of eleven weeks.

SUBJECT FIVE, an increase of 7,300 percent as a result of one exercise every fourteen days for a period of five months.

Impossible? I would have said so myself as recently as four years ago, but, as it happens, the last listed of the above five subjects was me. When first tested, my strength six degrees short of full extension of the lumbar spine produced an output of only four foot-pounds of torque; five months later, in the same position, I produced 296 foot-pounds of torque with the totally isolated muscles that extend the lumbar spine.

To say that we were surprised by the results is to put it mildly indeed, we were stunned.

It is also interesting to note that four out of the above five subjects had been using a Nautilus Lower-back Machine on a regular basis for periods varying from two to six years prior to the start of this isolated exercise." [2]

◄ The Nautilus Lower-back machine had a 250-pound weight stack that no one attempted during the seven years it sat in my gym. It was heavy . . . but heavy is relative. Subject Four (above) was MedX General Manager, Jim Flanagan who *could* lift the entire weight stack. To accommodate Jim's strength, Arthur built a machine with a 450-pound weight stack that likewise proved inadequate. Jim routinely performed the exercise in good form with two 200-pound men standing on the weight stack—a total of approximately 850 pounds. No one questioned his strength or effort when he was first tested on the MedX Lumbar Extension machine. His strength curve appeared "impressive," but there was nothing to compare it to—no norms, no ideal curve established. The surprise came when Jim re-tested at eleven weeks. He was fifteen times stronger, not fifteen percent. His 1,460 percent increase in strength in the final angle of full extension pointed to one thing only—muscle atrophy. Such a dramatic increase can ONLY occur when atrophy exists. Who would have guessed that Jim's lumbar strength entering the experiment was pitiful? He could lift 850 pounds on the Nautilus machine but was not strong when the large muscles of the hip were removed from the effort. Jim was strong somewhere, but it was not his lumbar extensors.

◄ On numerous occasions I played golf in Venezuela with an orthopedic back surgeon and twenty-year bodybuilder, Dr. Guillermo Bajares. He looked the part and had a long history of performing, among other exercises, weighted hyperextensions off the end of a bench. When my MedX Lumbar Extension machine arrived in Caracas I invited Dr. Bajares to test his strength. He promptly removed his tie, pumped his chest a few times and, judging by the color of his face, gave me a good effort. The results said otherwise. His strength was twenty percent below norms for men his age and size. Years of traditional low-back exercise had yielded few results.

◄ Steve Z. held nothing back. He entered my MedX facility in Coral Springs, Florida and introduced himself—for his age and weight—as "the current world-record holder in weightlifting." I didn't question it—his hamstrings and butt spoke for themselves. Steve was curious about "the machine that could measure back strength" and mentioned a pending competition. "Let's go," I said—the strongest man in the world was going to show me a thing or two. Not so: ONE, his strength was slightly below average compared to norms established in research; TWO, he fatigued quickly; THREE, his ideal protocol (according to research) was one minute of exercise every two weeks. Steve knew physiology and refused to comply. He came in once a week. After five sessions he demanded a re-test and once again held nothing back. Steve had lost eighteen percent strength because he was over-trained—once a week, as I suspected, was too much for back muscles that literally "couldn't stand much exercise." From that point on, Steve exercised once every two weeks for one minute. We retested following a number of sessions. This time he gained the eighteen percent he had lost and another twenty percent. By now three things were apparent: All of his competitive lifting and practice had little to no effect on the isolated strength of his lumbar extensors. Due to pelvic rotation, his efforts strengthened hip muscles; brief, infrequent and specific exercise is required to stimulate the lumbar muscles; and, the right tool is required for the task. You can't weigh yourself with a toaster.

◄ James Graves, Ph.D., conducted MedX Lumbar Extension research at the University of Florida in the late 1980's and early 1990's. When first tested for his fatigue characteristics (a muscle fiber-type test), Graves performed so many repetitions that he left Arthur Jones with a "perplexed look on his face." Jones thought Graves did not fully cooperate on his strength test—but Arthur was wrong. During every test that followed (about 100) Graves displayed unparalleled endurance. Immediately after *every* performance, he had *gained* strength—to Jones, a "genetic freak." Dr. Graves transferred to Syracuse University where he continued his research. In 1994 he tested the isolated low-back strength of sixteen elite male rowers from the collegiate team and compared the results to norms of untrained men the same size, age and weight (6'2", 190 pounds). According to Graves the rowers were *"marginally higher at full extension, but not statistically significant,"* which means if you walked into your local grocery store, found someone the same size, age and weight, and measured his back strength on the MedX machine, the result would be similar to that of the collegiate crew. Graves concluded, *"Rowing does not develop a significant amount of lumbar extension strength."*

◾ A MedX staff member took a series of muscle fiber-type tests on the Lumbar Extension machine to determine the fatigue rate of his low-back muscles. The results revealed a consistent loss of strength in the post-exercise test of 18%—indicative of an average mix of fast- and slow-twitch muscle fibers. On one occasion the subject performed the same test but substituted a Nautilus Lower-back machine (instead of MedX) for the exercise. The post-test revealed an average *increase* in strength of 2.5 percent throughout the range of motion with the exception of a slight decline in full extension. Eleven repetitions to muscle failure had no effect on his fresh-strength status which shows that *other* muscles were used during exercise on the Nautilus machine. Figures 4 and 5 of Chapter 18 represent the graphic results of his efforts.

◾ Gary Reinl volunteered for a MedX low-back test during "The Challenge of the Lumbar Spine" in New York City (1987)—Jones' formal introduction of the new tool. The test revealed an abnormal strength curve, a high rate of fatigue and poor recovery ability (typical of subjects with a predominance of fast-twitch muscle fibers). He decided to do something about it and immediately initiated a program of exercise on a Cybex Lower-back machine, three times per week. A stronger Reinl retested on the MedX machine four years later only to find that his strength had declined by twenty-two percent. More motivated, Gary trained for a year on a Nautilus Lower-back machine and, when re-tested on the MedX, registered no change. He then exercised for a full year on a second-generation Nautilus Lower-back machine only to find that he had further deteriorated. Despite progressively heavier weights on each machine, an awareness of his needs and plenty of hard work, the muscles that extended his spine *lost* strength for six years. Why? They were never stimulated. Traditional low-back exercise strengthens hip and rear-thigh muscles but does *not* access the muscles that extend the spine. *"So far,"* claimed Jones, *"we have found only two exceptions to that general rule: One, so-called 'hyper-extension' movements performed on a simple bench called a 'Roman Chair', and two, water-ski activities; but, in both cases, any resulting increases in lower-back strength are produced only near the fully-extended position of the movement."* [3]

Enough said. When it comes to full-range lumbar-extension strength gains, bodybuilding exercises don't cut it (ask Dr. Bajares), commercial gym machines don't do it (ask Gary Reinl and Jim Flanagan) and sports activities don't work (ask Steve Z. and the collegiate crew at Syracuse University). Why, then, do trainers insist on draping a client over a Swiss ball to do it? Arthur Jones was inactive when the Swiss-ball explosion occurred but an expression of his comes to mind (he would *not* have dignified a comparison): *". . . like comparing the Concord to an Ox cart."*

Test the low-back strength of any traditional "core" exerciser using a MedX Lumbar Extension machine, and I guarantee a poor result. And, if they exercise over time on any device that allows the pelvis to rotate (Swiss ball, bench, Nautilus or Cybex machine), I guarantee there will be NO strength change on a subsequent test, unless backwards counts.

The most important third of the core is clear: You CANNOT strengthen the muscles of the lumbar spine by traditional means.

Abdominal Muscles

There's better news with the abdomen: It can be strengthened. The question remains, "Does it need to be?" From the perspective that stronger muscles for sports or activities of daily living improve performance, the answer is, "Yes." From the perspective that strengthening a muscle group whose importance has been hyped, not proven, the answer is, "No." From that of strengthening minor muscles at the expense of major muscles, the answer is, "No." From that of strengthening a muscle group with exercises we despised in grade-school PT class, the answer is, "No." And, from the perspective of a trainer brought up to believe otherwise, the answer is a resounding, "NO."

Functional and sport-specific advocates disagree. They believe that abdominal muscles are vital to performance, low-back rehabilitation and muscle balance; that their importance has been proven by research and by the fact that everyone is strengthening them; that training time should be dedicated as much to minor as major muscle groups; and that the use of functional exercise and its tools (or none at all) is the most effective way to strengthen abdominal muscles.

Arthur Jones was called "a genius in body mechanics and exercise physiology" by the Ph.D.'s he worked with at the University of Florida. He didn't miss much—was thorough and honest. If Jones had perceived abdominal muscles as invaluable to corporal stimulation or performance, he would have declared so on the spot—and done something about it. But he saw nothing. He took a decade to develop an abdominal tool for Nautilus and did not include any with his MedX testing and rehabilitation equipment. The abdomen did *not* get his attention—which makes today's frenzy even more suspicious.

Years ago I was surprised by the sudden priority given to abdominal exercise: Trainees would start and end with abdominal movements and do little between. I was equally baffled by the priority afforded inferior resistance sources—bodyweight, pulleys, hanging straps and rubber balls.

If I performed abdominal exercise at all (and I do not), I'd prefer machines. Some of the early Nautilus models were excellent: They applied resistance to the muscles by placing elbows on separate pads and pushing downward. The version I owned fixed shins against pads and allowed the seat to simultaneously rotate upward. Later models left the seat in a fixed position. Both were effective because they allowed abdominal muscles freedom to perform their function—curl the torso toward the hips—and allowed hands to remain relaxed. Other models (and Arthur made several) applied resistance directly to the torso via a pad across the chest. Unfortunately, that style activated hip flexors which arched the torso (instead of flexing it) and bothered backs. If you overload an abdominal machine that applies resistance directly to the chest or front torso, you *will* hurt your back. But, if you have access to a good one, use it. It will save a trip to the floor—and worse—the return.

> You CANNOT strengthen the muscles of the lumbar spine by traditional means.

For every dozen grade-school exercises for the low back there must be 100 for the abdomen. Upper, lower, planks, twists, face-up, face-down, on the ball, off the ball, through dozens of angles and planes: If they invented as many variations for chest and/or biceps exercises, bodybuilders would never leave. Variety is trendy and abdominal exercise satisfies the primal instinct: *"There's fat around my belly—I need abdominal exercise."* Despite the fact that you cannot lose fat locally and that performing large-muscle-group exercise is more effective than small-muscle-group exercise for losing body fat, many people still believe that exercise "for the parts they need" is the way to go. So, in spite of honorable intentions, the abdominal frenzy will continue to have long-term appeal.

My back is about as strong as I can make it, but my abdomen is not. The imbalance would be of great concern to those who believe in "core" exercise and muscle balance. But I won't change. My back has been pain-free for decades and my golf handicap is as low as ever. Could I feel and perform better by working abdominals? Perhaps, but I prefer to prove a lot of people wrong.

Oblique Muscles

The sides of the core consist of muscles called "obliques." They bend laterally and twist which endears them to racquet sports, golf, basketball, volleyball, football, swimming, throwing, activities of daily living and to current trends in exercise—where their importance depends upon whom you ask. Arthur Jones recognized their value and spent fourteen years developing a rotary-torso machine that isolated the oblique muscles for the purpose of low-back rehabilitation.

Nonetheless, the torso-rotation machines found in gyms are among the worst-used. Jones built several models (Nautilus and MedX) that fixed the hips and allowed upper-body rotation but was never satisfied with the degree of muscle isolation. He later created a prototype that fixed the upper body while the lower body rotated—a version he never marketed. In the end there was no doubt about the isolation provided by his MedX medical device or its proper use. It's tough to abuse something when you can barely breathe.

Modern oblique training takes core exercise and adds a twist, which provides unlimited variety—nothing more. Dr. Fulton once witnessed a therapist attach latex tubing to the frame of a $60,000 MedX Torso Rotation machine to perform a standing version of the same. *"Like tying a horse to your car,"* he said, *"and pulling it around town."* To the therapist's credit, it *was* state-of-the-art tubing.

The point is this: If you need to strengthen a muscle, find the best tool and get the job done. Trainees have been brainwashed by functional advocates, become blind to reality or prefer the easy way out—which is never the most effective.

Conclusion

For two years I lived a few doors down the hall from legendary magician and illusionist, Doug Henning at McMaster University. It provided the opportunity to see plenty of magic before the "magic" of the Swiss ball was introduced.

I'm not opposed to strengthening any muscle and believe that strength improves performance if that muscle is involved. I object to the emphasis on "core" muscles at the expense of the more important larger muscle groups and object to the use of inferior equipment, especially when better is available.

So, don't waste your time and energy on the overused phrase, "the powerhouse." If you must strengthen your core: Perform one set of 8-12 repetitions on a MedX Lumbar Extension machine (once a week) and one set (twice a week) on best torso-rotation and abdominal machines you can find—a *total* of five minutes per session. If you have difficulty locating a MedX machine, visit **medxonline.com.** The larger medical versions are generally found in rehab centers but require a technician to put you in and drag you out. The smaller models located in gyms are self-serve but require set-up assistance.

Truth has a way of evading the field of exercise and core training is no exception. My opinion may lack the "magic" of the Swiss ball—*"the slick leading the blind"*—but it is closer to the truth.

REFERENCES

[1] Jones, A., *The Lumbar Spine, The Cervical Spine and The Knee: Testing and Rehabilitation*, MedX Corporation, Ocala, Florida, 8: 88, 1993.

[2] Fulton, M., M.D., "Lower-Back Pain: a New Solution For An Old Problem," 1988.

[3] Jones, A., *The Future of Exercise (1997 and Beyond)*, from The Arthur Jones Collection compiled by Johnson, B.D., Bodyworx Publishing.

CHAPTER 18

···

A Case for Low-Back Strength

T he short balding man gathered a handful of co-workers. *"I plan to build a machine that totally isolates muscle function,"* he announced. *"When I say something about a muscle, it will be 100% of that muscle, nothing less. The machine will take approximately six months to build at a cost of $200,000."* Deep down, he believed he could complete the task in three weeks for less than $10,000.

To add to the difficulty, he selected the muscles of the front thigh (quadriceps)—and later—those that extend the lumbar spine (erector spinae). It was January, 1972.

Arthur Jones was no stranger to challenge. In 1948 he began constructing an exercise tool to address the lagging development of his torso. Twenty-two years later he introduced a fifteen-foot long, six-foot wide and eight-foot high four-station device at the 1970 Mr. America contest in Culver City, California. "The Blue Monster" ushered in the era of Nautilus machines.

He began this project by modifying existing tools to test the strength of front and rear thighs, but it took more than a few weeks. *"An acceptable version of such a machine,"* he said, *"was not produced until April of 1991, nineteen years and three months after we started. Even a few months earlier, and after years of continuous work, it still appeared to be an impossible undertaking; every time we solved one problem we became aware of other, previously unsuspected problems."*

The development of a tool to isolate the spinal extensors proved equally complex. As he had done before, Jones applied a variable resistance directly to the working muscles—in this case, the upper torso as it extended through a full-range motion. The result—the Nautilus Lower-back machine—was the first of its kind to provide exercise for the muscles of the lumbar spine. *"I promise you,"* he wrote in his introductory article, *"If your lower back is out you won't care how big your arms are."* [1] He then attached a strain gauge to the device to explore the relationship between muscle strength and low-back pain.

In 1982 I purchased the Nautilus tool to complete my gym line, used it three times a week for four years to address two low-back surgeries and returned to Ocala to thank the inventor. His news was a shock: *"My back machine doesn't work."*

"When I designed that machine, I clearly understood that it provided exercise for both the hip and thigh muscles . . . but I believed that it also provided meaningful exercise for the lumbar-extensor muscles; an assumption that I now realize was wrong. The machine is misnamed, is in fact a hip and thigh machine, provides meaningful exercise only for the muscles of the buttocks and rear of the thighs." [2]

The machine allowed the pelvis to rotate which activated the large muscles of the hip . . . and more. It activated his competition. Following decades of research that supported Jones' contention, every major exercise-machine manufacturer made—and continues to make—a back machine that Arthur warned, *". . . will do nothing for the strength of lower-back muscles."*

Jones continued his quest to eliminate the contribution of hip muscles from the movement. How could he prevent the pelvis from rotating? Its upward rise and forward shift during torso extension led to sleepless nights as prototype after prototype failed. Finally, one caught his eye. Arthur successfully anchored the pelvis in a "stand-up" model. *"The pelvis did not rotate,"* he claimed, *"but it took two people to put you in and three to drag you out."* No one would return.

What led to the final solution struck like lightning: Why not use the femur (the upper-thigh bone that attaches to the pelvis) to *indirectly* prevent pelvic rotation? Illustrated below (Figure 1), Jones wedged the femur into the pelvis at an angle controlled by a small pad located above the knee. The force generated by a crank that moved the foot platform (A) toward the hips (in the direction of the arrows) prevented the pelvis from moving forward. The thigh-restraint belt (B) simultaneously provided a fulcrum to control the angle at which the femur contacted the pelvis and prevented the pelvis from rising during extension. Properly secured, the pelvis could not move forward and no longer rise. The problem appeared solved—but not for Jones. *"Believing that the pelvis is not moving during testing or exercise is not good enough,"* he said. *"You must* know *that the pelvis is not moving."* Proof was ultimately provided by a round, free-moving pad placed behind the pelvis (C). If the pelvis rotated one millimeter, the pad moved two—and any undesired movement could be eliminated by tightening the footboard and/or thigh-restraint adjustment. The significance of the degree of stability provided by the new device was yet to be determined.

> **Believing that the pelvis is not moving during testing or exercise is not good enough. You must *know* that the pelvis is not moving.**

Figure 1: **MUSCLE ISOLATION - PELVIC RESTRAINT**

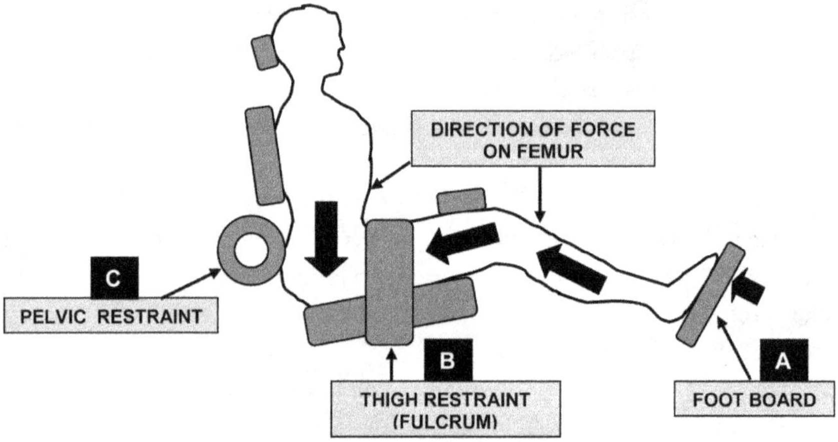

Fourteen years, 3,000 prototypes and $88 million later, Jones introduced his new device, the MedX Lumbar Extension machine at "The Challenge of the Lumbar Spine" in the Waldorf Astoria Hotel, New York City, October 8th and 9th, 1987. To advertize the event he published a full-page article in *The*

Washington Post, titled, *A Partial Solution for a Forty-Billion-Dollar Annual Problem for Industry, Insurance and Government— Screening for Lower Back Problems.* The statistical evidence from 10,000 lumbar evaluations was clear: "It appears that approximately thirty percent of a random group of people are at high risk of injury to the soft tissue in the area of the lumbar spine . . . while about ten percent have a genetic advantage that lowers the risk of injuries in this part of the body . . . about sixty percent do not have a similar advantage, but are well outside the high-risk category . . . These important differences, frequently critical differences, between individuals are produced by genetic factors that are not subject to change. With the use of proper, specific exercise, the lower-back strength can be greatly increased in almost any individual; and increasing the strength in the lumbar muscles will reduce the chances of injury. But subjects in the high-risk group will still be more likely to suffer from lumbar problems. Exercise will help, but cannot alter a genetic risk-factor."

The genetic risk factor was **muscle fiber-type**—essentially, a muscle's fatigue rate. "A recently-published study attempting to correlate lower-back strength with probability of lower-back injuries," said Jones, "found a negative relationship; the stronger subjects suffered more injuries. But they tested for the wrong factor; they should have tested for fiber type. The factor that made them strong also made them high-risk subjects for lower-back injuries."

According to Jones, a muscle with an average mix of fast- and slow-twitch fibers lost 2% strength per repetition. That is, ten repetitions of exercise to fatigue resulted in a strength loss of 20%, measured by pre- and post-exercise evaluations. Approximately 60% of subjects fatigued at this rate and were outside the high-risk category. Stronger-than-average subjects (30% of a random group) fatigued at a quicker rate and were at higher risk of injury in prolonged or repetitive tasks. Ten percent (10%) fatigued at a slower-than-average rate (exhibited low strength but high endurance) and were considered at low risk of back injury. Fiber-type cannot be altered by training but can be measured and exercised with an appropriate protocol. Fast-fatigue muscles, for example, can't stand much exercise, often have recovery issues and best respond to brief, infrequent stimulation.

Besides fiber-type, the MedX Lumbar Extension machine identified two additional risk factors associated with the muscles that extend the spine: ONE, **Specific** or **General** response to exercise; and TWO, **Chronic Disuse Atrophy**. The first dealt with how a muscle reacts to exercise, that is, does partial range-of-motion exercise result in partial-range fatigue and results (a SPECIFIC response) or full-range fatigue and results (a GENERAL response), as described and illustrated in Chapter 8. The difference could be determined from the slope of the strength curve—the relationship of peak strength in extension versus flexion. The top line of Figure 2 (below) represents the perfect relationship between strength in flexion versus strength in extension and the distribution of resistance to the working muscles (provided by the cam) *during* exercise on the MedX device—the Ideal Curve.

Figure 2:

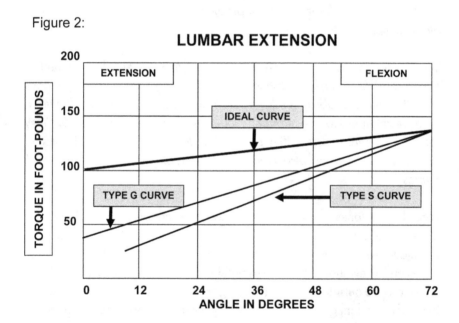

Those who exhibit a General response to exercise (Type G Curve) possess a 60% deficiency (compared to the Ideal) in their weakest position (left side of chart). Those exhibiting a Specific response (Type S Curve) feature an even greater deficiency in that position. A low level of strength in extension (compared to where it should or could be) increases the risk of back problems. According to Jones' studies and later confirmed by research, eighty percent (80%) of a random group of subjects exhibited a Specific response to exercise—were in the high-risk category. Fortunately, both curves (Specific and General) respond to isolated exercise by changing their shape in the direction of the Ideal Curve. And, proportionate strength throughout the range of motion reduces the risk of injury.

The final risk factor, **muscle atrophy**, surfaced during examination of the typical response to MedX lumbar exercise. Five decades of prior research demonstrated an average increase in strength of 20-30% after several months of training. Response to the MedX tool was unique and dramatic, and pointed in one direction—atrophy. If you put your arm in a cast for a month and take it out, you can increase its strength by several hundred percent because of its low initial level. That's what happened with use of the MedX machine. Exceptional and rapid strength increases were common in 90% of subjects after a twelve-week protocol.

Figure 3 (below) illustrates the three risk factors associated with the muscles that extend the lumbar spine and helps explain why—according to medical estimates—80% of people suffer from back pain in their lifetimes.

Figure 3: **RISK FACTORS FOR SPINAL INJURY**

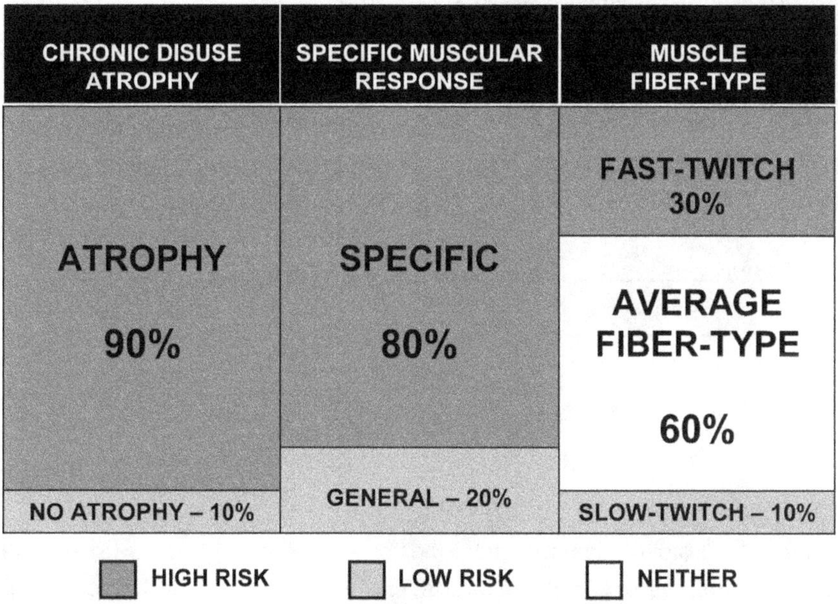

CHRONIC DISUSE ATROPHY	SPECIFIC MUSCULAR RESPONSE	MUSCLE FIBER-TYPE
ATROPHY 90%	SPECIFIC 80%	FAST-TWITCH 30%
		AVERAGE FIBER-TYPE 60%
NO ATROPHY – 10%	GENERAL – 20%	SLOW-TWITCH – 10%

■ HIGH RISK　　□ LOW RISK　　□ NEITHER

Jones tested the isolated low-back strength of five staff members, all of whom had used his Nautilus Lower-back machine for years. He was surprised when they all *exploded* in strength (as if they had done no prior exercise) and believed that the new device truly isolated and exercised the neglected muscles. To demonstrate the effect of (and need for) pelvic restraint, he subjected one of the five to a series of muscle-fatigue tests: a pre-exercise test of fresh strength, followed *immediately* by an intense exercise to muscle failure and *immediately* by a post-exercise test of exhausted strength. The difference between pre- and post-exercise tests would reveal the immediate, short-term effect of the exercise. The results of one of the fatigue tests are illustrated below.

Figure 4 demonstrates strength loss from a pre—(#1) and post—(#2) exercise test. When the subject performed exhausting exercise on a device that prevented pelvic rotation (MedX), he consistently lost 18-20% strength due to fatigue (a value confirmed by a number of similar tests).

Figure 4:

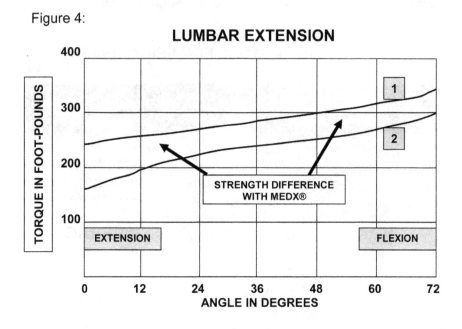

Figure 5 (below) demonstrates the same pre—(#1) and post—(#2) muscle-fatigue test with the exercise, on this occasion, performed on a

Nautilus Lower-back machine. As illustrated, there was no difference between the tests—NO strength loss as a result of performing exercise that allowed pelvic rotation (Nautilus).

The bad news: All current traditional low-back exercises allow pelvic rotation. When the pelvis rotates, the small muscles that extend the back DO NOT CONTRIBUTE TO—NOR BENEFIT FROM—THE EFFORT.

Figure 5:

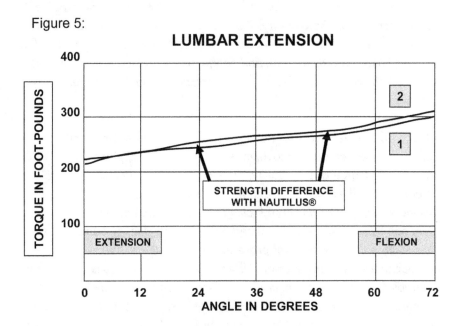

LUMBAR EXTENSION

Making it Official

To verify the effectiveness of his tool, Jones established the Center for Exercise Science at the University of Florida in Gainesville and watched from afar as study after study confirmed what his research already had. And he made it clear from the beginning: *"Let the chips fall where they may."* The research was relentless. *"By the end of this year (1987),"* he predicted, *"we should have completed testing of 30,000 subjects, and will test at least another 100,000 during 1988."*

The initial studies focused on the accuracy and reliability of the tool—and revealed the muscle's unique potential for strength gain. Subsequent studies established an efficient and effective exercise protocol (quantity, frequency, duration, etc.) and confirmed the need for pelvic stability during exercise and testing. The next step was to investigate the effect of strength on chronic back pain where one thing was apparent: You had better strengthen the right muscles.

"Weakness in the large muscles of the buttocks and legs is not the problem;" claimed Jones," *on the contrary, the strength of these muscles may be the source of the problem in lower-back injuries. When these larger and far stronger muscles produce a high and dangerous level of force that is imposed on the much weaker muscles of the lumbar area, then you frequently will have a problem."*

Arthur's device went beyond testing the strength and work-capacity of the lumbar muscles for pre-employment screening and job placement. *"With a very high degree of probability, the existence of a claimed injury to the lumbar area of the lower back can now be confirmed or refuted by a totally specific test of lumbar function; lacking any other confirmation, an existing injury can be proven . . . or a claimed but non-existent injury can be refuted. If an injury exists, the test will prove it; if not, the test will prove that too."* The machine was a lie detector. *"If you try to fake the results in an effort to establish a non-existent injury, the testing machine will catch you."* Yet, *"The test results of a co-operative subject will repeat themselves almost as closely as his finger prints."* How many billions of dollars would that save in health care?

The medical community believed (and still does) that a high percentage of back problems are muscular (or soft tissue) in nature—yet knows nothing about the muscles. *"Damage to the soft tissue in the region of the lumbar spine"*, claimed Jones, *"will seldom be revealed by an X-ray, may or may*

> **All current traditional low-back exercises allow pelvic rotation. When the pelvis rotates, the small muscles that extend the back DO NOT CONTRIBUTE TO - NOR BENEFIT FROM - THE EFFORT.**

not be detected by a CAT-scan or by Magnetic resonance Imaging . . . but almost certainly will be discovered by this test." (a pre-/post-exercise strength test on the MedX Lumbar Extension machine). He wasn't blowing smoke.

With momentum on his side, Jones established a second educational/ research center, this one at the University of California, San Diego, under the direction of Dr. Vert Mooney (a renowned orthopedic surgeon). At its peak the center treated 800 people per week to its twelve-week lumbar protocol. The volume of statistics hastened a conclusion concerning the effect of isolated exercise on chronic back pain. *"If you have been suggested for low-back surgery,"* declared Dr. Mooney, *"you would be crazy not to try the MedX Lumbar Extension machine (and its protocol) as a last resort."* It worked . . .

. . . but there were skeptics.

The second medical seminar I attended in Ocala, Florida (1996) was hosted by a Canadian engineer and medical doctor, Les Organ. Dr. Organ was a vocal advocate of isokinetic technology—motorized exercise and dynamic muscle testing in common use in rehabilitation clinics around the world. Jones hired Dr. Organ and gave him financial reign to build "the best isokinetic machine on the planet." And he did—a leg-extension machine (in eighteen months) at a cost of three million dollars (1980). At the time, Jones could prove beyond the shadow of a doubt that dynamic muscle testing and isokinetic technology was inaccurate and dangerous; and he stood at the doctor's side as they tested the new device. *"I told you so,"* was the redundant theme. Organ announced at the seminar that the information gleaned from dynamic testing on his *super* tool was an artifact. *"At best,"* he claimed, *"the measurement of force* (produced by the front thigh during dynamic testing) *is 100-200% in error."* And, *"At best, the angle to which the force corresponds is 40-60 degrees in error."* In other words, if a muscle registered a force of 100 units at an angle of 90 degrees, it may have been 300 units at 30 degrees or other random figures. This false information had misled medical and insurance communities for twenty years—and led to millions of rehabilitation treatments based on false information.

During every medical seminar, Jones ranted and raved about isokinetic technology, often pointing the finger at the leader in worldwide sales, Cybex®. One day someone in the crowd interrupted his soliloquy: *"Those are strong words, Arthur. Aren't you afraid they (Cybex) will sue?"* The reply was swift. *"I've been hoping they'll sue me for 20 years. When we go to court, it will take three minutes to prove that one and one is two—not eight."* Cybex wouldn't touch him and eventually, as did others, phased out the product. Unfortunately, the majority of medical facilities across the nation had isokinetic technology and paid plenty for it ($50,000). They were not pleased upon hearing the truth.

The machine that *Business Week* described as *"a Lazyboy® recliner designed by the Marquis de Sade"* could test the strength of, and provide exercise for, the isolated muscles that extend the spine. Along the way, Jones discovered that the test output was influenced by, among other things, the size of the subject. More specifically, force output was *diminished* during muscle testing by the effect of gravity in flexion (seated with chest near thighs; Figure 6, A, below), and *increased* by gravity in extension (torso extended back; Figure 6, C). The illustration that follows demonstrates the compensation required during the test of a 200-pound, six-foot tall male at 48° of flexion and 24° of extension. Jones counterweighted the subject's torso weight throughout the range of motion and double-checked the accuracy of his efforts by developing a machine that tested strength *without* the effect of gravity. Once secured in the MedX Lumbar Lateral machine, the subject was rotated as if on a barbeque so that test efforts were registered in a horizontal rather than vertical plane. Test results *with gravity* were then compared to those *without gravity* to confirm the accuracy of the counterweight system.

> **If you have been suggested for low-back surgery, you would be crazy not to try the MedX Lumbar Extension machine (and its protocol) as a last resort.**

Figure 6: **EFFECT OF TORSO MASS ON TORQUE OUTPUT**

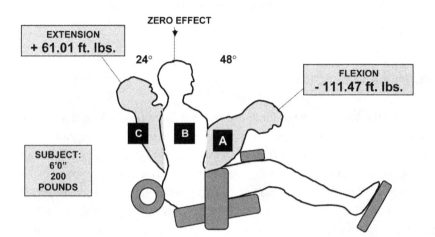

The effort paid off. In the early 1990's Arthur paraded a group of Asian businessmen through our certification classroom at the University of Florida to reveal the scope of his project, unaware that they were skeptical of his counterweight system. The group purchased a machine and performed a meticulous two-year evaluation that established a high degree of accuracy throughout the entire range of motion.

At some point, the MedX Lumbar Extension machine was nominated for a Nobel Prize in medicine.

Jones ignored the accolades and continued work on a tool to isolate the muscles of the front thigh—a challenge that introduced seven problems beyond those of the lumbar machine. He completed the task in twenty years at a cost of approximately $120 million.

On one visit to Ocala, Arthur took me on a private tour of his manufacturing facility located on the far side of his jumbo-jet runway. The first lumbar extension machine was used in his daily medical presentations; the second, in research at the University of Florida. The frame of the third stared me in the face. Jones paused to explain why the underlying structure was double that of a Nautilus machine—a staff member saw the original frame bend as the lap belt was secured.

The heavy, intimidating, expensive device caught my attention. Following a long history of back issues, I had to give it a go. The decision may have been my finest hour.

Oh, Those Water Skiers . . .

Dr. Michael Fulton, the orthopedic representative for MedX, was the official physician of the US Water-Ski Team and had access to eighteen of the top twenty skiers in the world. When he tested the elite group for the isolated strength of their spinal extensors, they exhibited a unique pattern. Unlike the majority of subjects who demonstrated greater strength in flexion than extension (illustrated by Figures 2, 4 and 5, above), the professional skiers possessed greater strength in extension than flexion—a product of their activity. Water skiers resist the pull of boats all day by leaning back. Yet, other professional athletes who extend their low backs during the execution of their activities (rowers, weight lifters, etc.) did *not* exhibit the same effect—and logically so. Weight lifters and rowers are exposed to greater resistance in their respective efforts when their torsos are in a flexed position. An increase in leverage and the effect of momentum expose the working muscles to less work in extension. Water-skiers on the other hand battle a sustained resistance in extension throughout their performance—and failure to maintain that posture results in a wet landing.

When the elite skiers were exposed to isolated exercise on the MedX device, their strength increased at both ends (in flexion *and* extension) and their strength curves slowly conformed to the Ideal (Figure 2). The ideal relationship of strength in flexion versus extension (1.4:1) was first established by Jones and reflected in the cam that applied resistance to the working muscles. Use of the machine forced subjects to adopt proportionate lumbar strength at every angle of movement—his greatest legacy.

> **The ideal relationship of strength in flexion versus extension (1.4:1) was first established by Jones and reflected in the cam that applied resistance to the working muscles.**

Research

Below are samples of conclusions from research that featured the MedX Lumbar Extension machine:

Strength Evaluation

"Objective evaluation of isolated lumbar extension strength is limited by the inability to stabilize the pelvis. Without stabilization, buttocks and hamstring muscles overshadow the smaller, weaker lumbar extensors." [3]

"Lumbar extension strength was clearly shown to be strongest in full flexion rather than mid range which is in contrast to what is found in the literature." [3] Preceding studies and literature reflected measurements that included contributions from the large muscles of the hip.

"These data show the lumbar extension machine to be highly reliable and specific for quantification of lumbar extension strength." [3]

Chronic Disuse Atrophy

"The magnitude of gain shown by the training group reflects the low initial trained strength of the lumbar extensor muscles. These data indicate that when the lumbar area is isolated through pelvic stabilization, the isolated lumbar extensor muscles show an abnormally large potential for strength increase." [4] (in this study, a 102% increase in extension and 42% increase in flexion)

Figure 7 (below) demonstrates the collective results produced by the first group of subjects to use a Medx Lumbar Extension machine for prolonged exercise. The grey columns (left side at each angle) represent the average static strength of the isolated back muscles measured *before* an exercise protocol that lasted from ten to twenty-seven weeks. The black columns (right side at each angle) represent strength levels attained *after* the protocol. Most subjects had a two-to-six-year history on the Nautilus Lower-back machine.

The average increase in the level of peak torque (strength) in flexion (right side of chart) was 87%, while the average in extension (left side) was 686%. The average overall strength increase throughout the range of motion was 142%. The MedX machine was used infrequently: at most, once a week; at least, once every two weeks. The subject who exercised for twenty-seven weeks performed only thirteen exercises and produced an increase in extension of 877%. The average time per exercise was brief—less than two minutes.

It was obvious that very little exercise was required to produce "exceptional" strength results with the muscles that extend the lumbar spine. It was equally obvious that too few took notice.

Figure 7: **STRENGTH GAINS**

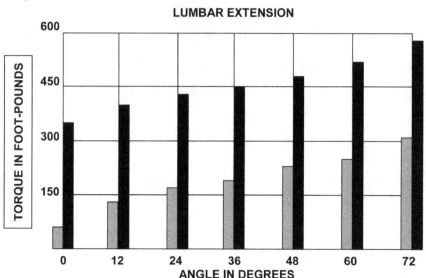

The average increase in the level of peak torque in flexion was 87%, while the average in extension was 686%. The average overall strength increase throughout the range of motion was 142%.

Training Frequency

". . . a training frequency as low as 1 X /week provides an effective training stimulus for the development of lumbar extension strength. Improvements in strength noted after isometric training suggest that isometric exercise provides an effective alternative for developing lumbar strength." [5] This study compared different training frequencies: 1x/wk, 2x/wk, 3x/wk, 1x/2 wks and isometric (a static muscle test at seven different angles, 1x/ wk). No significant difference was detected among the frequencies.

"These findings show that isometric lumbar extension torque (strength) increases occur mainly within the first 12 weeks of training, although additional gains in the more extended positions can be expected when training is continued through 20 weeks." [6]

". . . training once every other week or once per week is as effective as training twice per week for increasing isometric lumbar extension torque over 20 weeks." [6]

Strength Maintenance

"These findings indicate that isometric lumbar extension strength can be maintained for up to 12 weeks with a reduced frequency of training as low as once every 4 weeks when the intensity and the volume of exercise are maintained." [7]

Figure 8 (below) illustrates the staying power of specific exercise for the lumbar spine. The black columns (right side at each angle) represent the average strength level of a large group of subjects following a twelve-week program of specific exercise. The grey columns (left side at each angle) represent strength following an additional twelve weeks of training using a frequency of one exercise every four weeks.

There was no change in strength in the first half of the range of motion (right side of chart), a 1% increase at mid-range and a 7% decrease in extension (left side of chart). Having increased the strength of the spinal muscles with specific exercise, very little in the way of additional exercise is required to maintain a peak level of strength.

Figure 8: **STRENGTH MAINTENANCE**

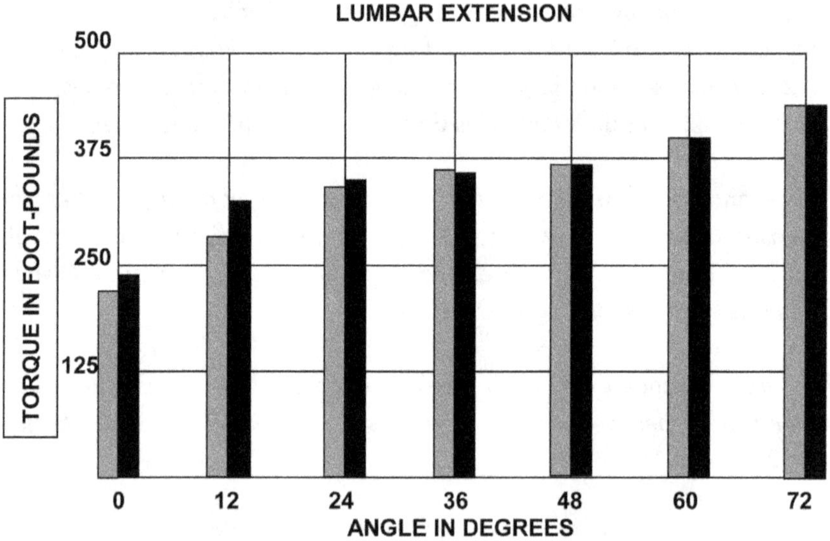

LUMBAR EXTENSION

The same study (above) was reported in *Medicine and Science in Sports and Exercise* (1990) with this summary: *"These findings: 1) extend previous research indicating that low frequency training is effective for increasing low back extensor strength. This is in contrast to what is shown when training other muscle groups; 2) reflect the atrophied state of the lumbar extensor muscles; 3) show that lumbar extension strength increases occur mainly within the first 12 weeks of training, although additional gains in the extended positions can be expected when training is continued through 20 weeks; 4) indicate that changes in peak strength are not indicative of changes throughout the lumbar extensor range-of-motion."*

One thing was apparent: The muscles that extend the lumbar spine are unique in their response to exercise—do not require much to attain peak strength and very little to maintain. The official protocol established by research at the University of Florida appeared too good to be true: twice a week for the first month; once a week for the next two months; one exercise per month to maintain. Its mention elicits disbelief, yet its results cannot be matched by other means, as follows:

Figure 9 (below) represents a research study[8] to determine the effect of training on commercial low-back machines to the development of isolated lumbar-extension strength. Seventy seven (77) healthy, normal subjects were tested for isometric low-back strength on a MedX Lumbar Extension machine and randomly divided into four groups. One group trained on the Nautilus Lower-back machine; one on the Cybex Eagle Low-back machine, one on the MedX machine and one not at all (Control Group; Curve #2). The training groups performed one exercise per week for twelve weeks and all groups tested their isometric strength at seven angles on the MedX device following the training period.

EFFECT OF TRAINING WITH PELVIC STABILIZATION ON LUMBAR EXTENSION STRENGTH

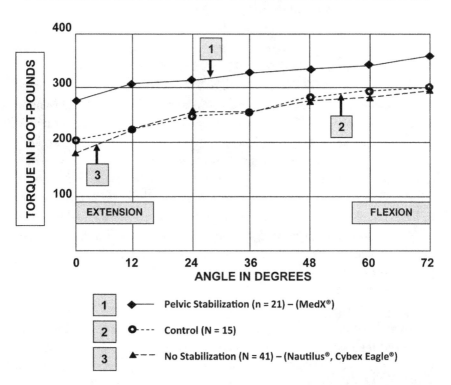

Both the Nautilus and Cybex Eagle groups showed no change in isolated lumbar extension strength at any of the measured angles and their results were combined into a "No Stabilization" group (Curve #3) for comparative purposes. The MedX group (Curve #1) showed a significant increase in isometric strength at each angle throughout the range of motion. An interesting observation in the study was the increase in dynamic strength (weight lifted) in ALL of the training groups.

The implications are clear: ONE, Pelvic stabilization is necessary to elicit a training effect in the lumbar extension muscles (the dynamic strength increases recorded in the Nautilus and Cybex groups were likely a training effect of the muscles that extend the hip—glutes and hamstrings); and TWO, the degree of pelvic stabilization provided by commercial low-back machines is inadequate to isolate the lumbar area and stimulate a response in the targeted muscles.

A Miner Problem

No one knew more firsthand than the Western Energy Company: Strip mining is tough on backs. The 1991-1993 US Department Interior Bureau of Mines reported 1.09 back injuries per 200,000 employee hours worked in strip mines. The nine-year average at Western's Rosebud Coal Mine in Colstrip, Montana was 2.94. On three occasions the government advised Western to implement an accident-reduction program. One state worker's compensation specialist was blunt. *"If we were a private insurer, we would give notice of cancellation. However, since we are the insurer of last resort, we can only continue to raise your premiums in relation to your loss ratio. In time, you will become non-competitive and fail as a business."* In July of 1992 Western Energy hired a new safety coordinator, Pat Rummerfield, who organized a trip to Ocala, Florida and persuaded the company to purchase the MedX device.

The program began in August, 1993 with thirty volunteer employees. By year's end, 180 workers were involved in a twenty-week protocol. The group increased their isolated low-back strength between 54-104%, and 80% of workers reported a reduction in pain perception. Forty percent (40%) were pain free. More importantly, the average worker's compensation liability of

$14,430.00 per month (the average for forty months *before* the arrival of the MedX tool) was reduced to a *total* of $389.00 for nine months following its use. From August 2, 1993 through March 31, 1994 the incidence of injury was .52 per 200,000 employee hours worked (with one back injury report). Among non-exercising workers the incidence remained high at 2.55 (with four reported injuries). Only two workers dropped out of the program. Besides its resounding success with the spine, *"The Lumbar Extension machine,"* according to Rummerfield, *"had a greater positive impact upon 'how employees perceived their employer' than any other programmatic activity preceding it."*

The MedX machine wiped out Western Energy's problem—while today's trainers insist on the use of a Swiss Ball and bodyweight exercises to get the job done.

A Medical Problem

Dr. Brian Nelson, an orthopedic physician from Minnesota, had heard it many times before: *"We've tried everything with this patient. He needs an operation."* Dr. Nelson introduced 38 patients (that physicians in his area had abandoned) to the MedX Lumbar Extension machine's official three-month protocol of brief, infrequent exercise. To the dismay of his peers, he published the results of his efforts in the January, 1999 edition of *Archives of Physical Medicine and Rehabilitation*. Thirty-five of the thirty-eight patients did NOT require surgery and the average of twenty-one MedX sessions saved more than a few backs. MedX therapy was $1,995.00; a single surgery, $60-160,000. The study was not "official" research (it lacked a control group and a randomized selection of participants, both of which were impractical in private practice) but the results were impressive. *"It does not prove,"* concluded Dr. Nelson, *"that increased strength prevents surgery. The study does suggest that certain people can avoid surgery, which is good news."* The outcomes were verified at follow-up intervals averaging sixteen months.

> More importantly, the average worker's compensation liability of $14,430.00 per month (the average for 40 months *before* the arrival of the MedX tool) was reduced to a *total* of $389.00 for nine months following its use.

A Personal Problem

My personal results were equally impressive. I underwent two lumbar surgeries by the age of thirty-two and suffered two major crises shortly thereafter. Fortunately, the neurosurgeon decided not to go back in all of this in Venezuela. I partnered with a gym member—a Nautilus devotee who followed the work of Arthur Jones—to purchase the MedX Lumbar Extension machine and establish a rehabilitation center in Caracas (1988). I could not afford another mistake and followed the protocol verbatim. In twenty weeks I was pain-free and began to wean myself from the once-a-week protocol by performing one set of approximately ten to fifteen repetitions every two weeks for several months, every three weeks for several months and settled on a once-a-month frequency as suggested by research. I have maintained my strength and pain-free status for twenty-four years with very little exercise. The muscles are truly unique in their response.

A General Problem

Despite the success of the MedX tool, most trainers are unaware of its existence or continue to ignore the facts. In the meantime, the powers-to-be have all but destroyed the value of muscle isolation, discredited the use of machines in general, ignored everything related to the work of Arthur Jones and replaced it with a ten-cent solution. I hope they're proud.

Some of the problems related to its lack of recognition extend beyond the scope of exercise. Research hasn't helped. *"MedX spinal therapy has amassed impressive research results,"* claimed one scientist, *"but little name recognition."* Research publications insist on equipment-manufacturer neutrality. They typically mention the manufacturer's name once and often fail to identify what produced the "good" result. *"MedX training indicates a stabilized pelvis, torso-mass counterbalance, isometric test points over a full or pain-free range of movement and several other innovative features exclusive to MedX equipment."* MedX testing and exercise are unique.

The press hasn't helped. In a *New York Times* report on Dr. Nelson's study (above), MedX therapy was identified as "weight lifting." When weight lifting or weight training is deemed effective in the treatment of chronic back pain, it triggers images of exercises that do *not* strengthen spinal extensors and might—in some cases—add to the problem. Misreporting can be a great disservice.

The ultimate insult was provided by the medical community: MedX was perceived a threat. Dr. Nelson co-authored a review of literature published in the January, 1999 edition of *Medicine and Science in Sports and Exercise* that represented an historical perspective of exercise related to spine care. *"Strengthening exercises,"* he stated, *"were initially used for physical therapy rather than general conditioning."* Somewhere down the line things changed. *"A review of 'modern' spine care over the past 30 years shows that these early concepts were abandoned in favor of passive modalities that predominantly treat symptoms."* The efficacy of passive modalities lacks scientific evidence; the efficacy of MedX treatment does not.

When all research was on the table, 80% of patients with chronic back pain (regardless of diagnosis) reported a reduction in pain perception after a twelve-week MedX protocol. Thirty to thirty-three percent (30-33%) became pain free. The success of the treatment prompted Arthur Jones to state toward the end of his career: *"If and when the government ever takes any meaningful steps in the direction of sanity, which I doubt, it could come to pass that all cases of lower-back pain will be treated first with MedX machines, that any other treatment will be prohibited until and unless MedX treatment has been tried and has failed. A simple federal law to that effect would save the people in this country a minimum of $80,000,000,000.00 a year."*

I have repeatedly declared: *"The MedX Lumbar Extension machine is the ONLY way to meaningfully access the muscles that extend the lumbar spine from a strength perspective."* And it's not because it's MedX and not because it was created by Arthur Jones. It's because the machine does not allow the pelvis to rotate during exercise. That's the key. To believe the pelvis is not rotating by focus or by will is not enough. You must literally hammer it down and KNOW that it is not moving. With the MedX tool you will KNOW: A blind man can detect pelvic rotation if you are properly secured.

As a result of the above, the reception to Jones' efforts has cooled. The number of rehabilitation clinics around the nation using MedX medical machines has diminished. Fewer gyms feature the exercise version and the corporation is in shambles. I have been fortunate to work in facilities that featured one or the other because the owner built his or her business around it. Many current fitness establishments do not offer a MedX lumbar machine because they "already have a back machine," are unaware of the difference or are not willing to pay the price. I recently worked in a North Carolina facility that featured the exercise version—backed in a corner where it sat for four years, cob-webs and all.

And what did clients use to strengthen their low backs during that time? Probably the same dog-and-pony exercises employed before the MedX era—bridges, hyperextensions, Swiss balls and other things that are USELESS for their intended purpose. And why do they still play a role in current training regimens? Is there no one bold enough to admit, *"My machine doesn't work?"* Is there something at stake, or something I've missed?

I'd like to believe that it's ignorance. Most trainers (especially those new to the field) are unaware of the MedX Lumbar Extension machine and its history, have never read related research and simply don't know a thing about it. But some do, and if you've read this far—you may be among that minority.

To me, there are two sides of the coin—and only one can be corrected.

HEADS: For those willing to learn, the MedX Lumbar Extension machine *test* protocol identifies the following:

- Three muscular risk factors associated with low-back pain: Specific response to exercise, muscle fiber-type and atrophy.
- A pain-free and functional range of motion.
- The strength of isolated lumbar extensor muscles at every angle through a full range of motion. It then compares strength and range-of-motion statistics to norms (age, sex and bodyweight) and ideal values (to distinguish weaknesses and abnormalities).
- An optimal exercise protocol to strengthen the muscles.
- False claims of low-back problems—fraud.

Its *exercise* protocol can achieve the following:

- Increase functional range of motion.
- Establish proportionate and full-range strength.
- Modify strength curves to approximate the Ideal.
- Reduce or eliminate pain perception in chronic cases.
- Address the root cause of most low-back problems—lack of muscle strength.

TAILS: For those not willing to learn, ask yourself the following . . .

If muscle isolation is so "non-functional," why is it absolutely essential to the strengthening of the most important muscles you have?

As someone once said, *"If you want to lead the orchestra, you must turn your back to the crowd."*

REFERENCES

[1] Jones, A., *"The Most Important Area of the Body? Featuring the Lower-Back Machine,"* Nautilus Magazine Supplement: 1982).

[2] Jones A., The Lumbar Spine, Sequoia Communications, 36, 1988.

[3] Graves, J.E., Pollock, M.L., *Quantitative Assessment of Full Range-of-Motion Lumbar Extension Strength*, Spine, 15: 289-294, 1990.

[4] Pollock, M.L., Leggett, S.H., Jones, A., Fulton, M., *Effect of Resistance Training on Lumbar Extension Strength*, The American Journal of Sports Medicine, 17 (5): 624-29, 1989.

[5] Graves, J.E., Pollock, M.L., Foster, D., Leggett, S.H., Carpenter, D.M., Vuoso, R., Jones, A., *Effect of Training Frequency and Specificity on Isometric lumbar Extension Strength*, Spine, 15 (6): 504-509, June 1990.

6 Carpenter, D.M., Graves, J.E., Pollock, M.L., Leggett, S.H., Foster, D., Holmes, B., Fulton, M.N., *Effect of 12 and 20 Weeks of Resistance Training on Lumbar Extension Torque Production*, Physical Therapy, 71 (8): 580-588, 1991.

7 Tucci, J.T., Carpenter, D.M., Pollock, M.L., Graves, J.E., Leggett, S.H., *Effect of Reduced Frequency of Training and Detraining on Lumbar Extension Strength*, Spine, 17 (12), December, 1992.

8 Graves, J.E, Webb, D.C., Pollock, M.L., Matkozich, J., Leggett, S.H., "Effect of Training with Pelvic Stabilization on Lumbar Extension Strength," Int. J Sports Med., 11: 403, 1990.

CHAPTER 19

Variety: Much Ado About Nothing

G ood form and high intensity are vital to the production of results from exercise. Yet, the vast array of "new" offerings that suddenly appear in fitness establishments with alarming frequency might lead you to believe that variety should be added to the list. Variety can affect progress only when the quality and intensity of the "new" is equal to or surpasses the "current" — which is not often the case. The "new" generally represents more hype than substance.

One thing I've learned in this field: If everyone heads West, you'd better go East — and quick.

Cross-Training

The terms "cross-training" and its sidekick "muscle confusion" have flooded the exercise landscape with more confusion than they're worth — which may have been the intent. *"Dazzle them with footwork"* has always played a large and profitable role in exercise.

At first glance, cross-training systems (P90X®, CrossFit®, Extreme Training®, Insanity® Training and whatever follows) revolve around intensity. They, ONE, introduce ways to make exercise more difficult using little or no equipment (What's the hardest way to perform a push-up or work the abdominals sequentially?); and TWO, minimize time between exercises which increases the overall effect of the stimulus. Both factors — harder exercise and decreased rest between efforts—are assets, but not new. They were staples of Nautilus training thirty-five years ago. That's where the similarity ends.

Intensity requires recovery, and recovery spells efficiency. Cross-training systems are none of the above. In 1977 Ellington Darden outlined in his book, *Strength Training Principles* a full-body Nautilus workout of Miami-Dolphin running-back, Mercury Morris that lasted thirteen minutes and six seconds. Every exercise was supervised and pushed (to ensure proper form and intensity) and workouts were performed no more than three times per week (a weekly total of less than forty minutes). During the workout the average rest afforded Morris between efforts was thirteen seconds. That's efficient.

Jones applied the same concepts to Boyer Coe's training at the Nautilus complex in 1983. When I arrived that year to purchase equipment, Coe was performing one set of eight exercises (sixteen minutes) twice a week. More exercise than that, according to Jones, left Mr. Universe in an *over-trained* state. That's efficient.

Why then, do cross-training programs insist on an hour of exercise (or more) each day, five to six days a week? Properly performed, no one *requires* or *can stand* (recover from) that much exercise—which leads to one conclusion: The recommended exercise is *not* properly performed.

In spite of the obvious and in the face of claimed efficiency, "muscle confusion" programs advocate exercise on most days, if not every day. Or they recommend something less active (but something nonetheless) on "off days." They rationalize their stance by performing different activities or by training distinct muscle groups each day—the confusion factor—when the weight of scientific evidence suggests "NO" to strength training (or other forms of strenuous physical activity) on consecutive days. One study compared running times and strength gains of track-and-field athletes using different training schedules. Group A lifted weights Monday, Wednesday and Friday, and ran for time Tuesday, Thursday and Saturday. Group B performed both activities the same day (3X/wk) and rested the next, a formula that produced superior strength gains *and* running times. Athletes in Group A kept recovery at bay by performing activity on what should have been an "off" day; whereas athletes in Group B shocked their systems more thoroughly on "exercise" days and recovered better on "off" days.

Cross-training and split-training programs do not allow sufficient rest and recovery between workouts. Arthur Jones often challenged bodybuilders who trained everyday "in parts" (and most did) with the following: *"Sleep tonight with your left eye open and tomorrow night with your right, and tell me how you do."* My challenge was similar, *"Did you eat lunch today for your calves or sleep last night for your shoulders?"* And, I once revealed my "training secret" to an aspiring bodybuilder: *"I split my body in half—trained the left half yesterday, the right half today."* The silence was deafening. He had never heard such stupidity (nor I), but it was the same stupid thing he was doing and claimed, "Everyone else was doing." Everyone once believed the world was flat.

I was close to believing the same on May 31ˢᵗ, 2008, when three men in their late-twenties entered the fitness center of the Lake Toxaway Country Club in North Carolina and asked for a skipping rope that we did not have. Upon return from a local hardware store, they promptly downloaded a workout from the internet and began to educate me on the virtues of "CrossFit."

I witnessed the brief, intense effort from the front row and found it hard to believe that anyone could create something that stupid, harder to believe that anyone would do it and hardest to believe that there was a pot of gold at the end of that rainbow. Every move was explosive—the routine laden with impact and the potential for injury.

To illustrate that potential, Jones once instructed a group of medical doctors during a conference to press a closed fist against a cinder-block wall as hard as they could for ten seconds. When they completed the task, he asked them to pull the fist back a few inches and punch the wall as hard as they could. Fortunately, the physicians had enough common sense to realize that the impact of hitting the wall would create "issues." Arthur then

---

Properly performed, no one *requires* or *can stand* (recover from) that much exercise.

explained that the force of the punch would actually be *less* than the press because muscles would not have enough time to recruit all of their fibers. Less force means less potential for injury, yet the addition of impact would have magnified the forces to high and dangerous levels.

Unfortunately, common sense did not prevail that day at Lake Toxaway. Curly, Larry and Moe jumped around like kangaroos for fifteen to twenty minutes and finished like a trio of snorting Clydesdales in an empty gym. Their cardiovascular effort may have indeed flattened the earth—but not much else. *"Enjoy it while you can,"* I thought. *"Joint systems comes with a limited warranty."* Men must do what men must do.

The *appeal* of cross-training programs may relate to the following:

1. By comparison, free-weight and machine training is boring. This "looks" more exciting, dynamic and "macho"—at least during the infomercials.
2. Trainees believe that performing a variety of activities (strength, endurance, agility, balance, power, interval work, etc.) makes them more rounded as an athlete or person.
3. Many professional teams train this way—and the public wants to train like the pros.
4. You can exercise "at home" with no special equipment. The system is portable.
5. The TV trainees appear to achieve higher heart rates and sweat more than viewers during their typical workouts. Therefore, it must be better.
6. "Before-and-after" testimonials convince trainees that they can do it *and* achieve similar results.
7. The variety of training may produce muscle soreness, and trainees falsely equate soreness with effectiveness. Muscle soreness is a function of "different"—not "better."
8. Intense muscle work can activate the cardiovascular system and improve body composition—an all-in-one approach.
9. Clever marketing has attracted major sponsors. The CrossFit Games, for example, are funded by Reebok® and identify "The Fittest on Earth."® But if you think you can't be more fit than CrossFit, you have a short memory (this generation has no memory). From

1970-74, *no one* completed the twelve-exercise Nautilus circuit at company headquarters. Ellington Darden was present for most of those workouts and claimed it wasn't close. No one lasted more than a few minutes with Arthur Jones, which makes "Fit" and "hard" relative.

The *non-appeal* of such programs may relate to the following:

1. If you are not "up" for hard work, don't start. High intensity, not muscle confusion, drives the program, and most people are not willing to work hard. If history is any indication, its difficulty may lead to its demise.

2. The quality of movement is poor—in some cases dangerous—due to explosive exercise speed. The theory that "fast" exercise recruits fast-twitch (powerful) muscle fibers is false. Research demonstrates that neither the load nor speed of movement determine fiber recruitment. Intensity is the trigger: *"The evidence suggests that individuals should be encouraged to train to momentary muscular failure, as this appears to maximize muscle-fiber recruitment and, according to most of the research to date, will maximize gains in strength and power."* [1] To the surprise of many, strength, power and momentary muscle failure can be safely achieved by the performance of slow, controlled movements.

3. If strength protects you from injury, full-range strength protects you more. Muscle-confusion programs fail to provide full-range exercise—and worse. The adherence to "explosive" speed and impact may one day prevent you from moving at all.

4. Positive changes in body-composition are due more to the dietary guidelines that accompany the program than the program itself. Without nutritional modification results are slow. But the implication is clear: If you bounce around like an idiot, you produce *this* result.

5. Expect a loss in flexibility unless a stretching regimen accompanies the program.

6. The skills learned in performing a variety of activities (boxing, kick-boxing, agility drills, power-lifting, etc.) are specific. If you improve at one activity—*and you will with practice*—it does not

make you a better overall athlete. It makes you better at that particular activity.

7. Hard to believe, but you can get fit, just as fit or more fit in less time and in a safer manner.

Cross-training attempts to shatter the boredom of traditional training and provide athletes an edge. Professional football has been historically vulnerable to that search. In the early 1970's Alvin Roy introduced the NFL to what Arthur Jones described as *"one of the worst outrages ever associated with the field of exercise"*—explosive training. Around that time, Roy visited Nautilus headquarters in Lake Helen. *"I initially assumed that he was simply stupid,"* said Jones, *"that he really believed what he was telling people."* Arthur was wrong. He visited a "training camp" supervised by Roy and found him doing everything but "explosive training" in an effort to not hurt anyone. He wasn't doing much to help anyone either. Roy later admitted that he was *"well aware of the dangers from explosive exercises but still promoted them as gospel because 'that was what coaches wanted to hear.'"* Hard to tell who was more stupid—Roy or the coaches? Nonetheless, it stuck and the NFL has been neck-deep in explosive nonsense since. The pile grew when someone convinced coaches that power-lifting movements were the key to power on the field. Then came agility and resistance drills (dragging tires and parachutes), balance drills and, last but not least, dance lessons. Stupidity has no limit. The strength gained in the performance of these tasks may translate into something of value. But the performance of agility, power and balance drills, and running-resistance activities does not increase agility, power or balance. They serve to demonstrate those qualities but have no *other* value, with one exception. Dance lessons NFL players took decades ago might help them in the end zone AFTER the touchdown.

TRX

The value of exercise should be judged by the quality of resistance and the range of motion over which the resistance is effective. Despite its popularity, TRX training fails on both counts—by applying straight-line force to rotational movement. The only thing that counts in strength training is the vertical movement of resistance directly against the pull of gravity. Anything but vertical lessens the effect of gravity and the effectiveness of the exercise.

With few exceptions, the black and yellow TRX straps that hang from gym ceilings provide resistance in an arc that rarely travels vertically. As a result, the effective strength curve (the application of resistance to the working muscles) is never correct, and often, the reverse of what it should be. For example, in the starting position of the TRX chest press (with arms fully extended and chest muscles fully contracted), the resistance (body weight) is at its minimum. Lowering the chest to a position of full stretch near the floor increases the resistance to its highest level—where shoulders are most vulnerable to injury and working muscles, weakest. The effective resistance is the opposite of what it should be. When a muscle is fully contracted the resistance should be at its peak, or at least adequate, to activate as many muscle fibers as possible.

The same deficiency applies to TRX pulling motions. During the row and regardless of foot placement, resistance is greatest when muscles are stretched and weakest when they are contracted—again, the opposite of ideal. Close your eyes as you perform any TRX exercise and tell me what you feel: A challenge when muscles are stretched and little when they are contracted.

Similar to the Universal® machine of the 1960's, TRX straps allow access to a variety of movements but most lack quality. Their difficulty lies in the instability inherent in the execution—a deterrent to the acquisition of strength. The working muscles spend most of their time and energy balancing the body and perfecting the skill which detracts from the goal of gaining strength. And worse: Trainers and trainees often confuse strength and skill gain. As things get easier with TRX movements, everyone assumes they are getting stronger when the bulk of improvement relates to skill.

To add: Bodyweight is a poor source of resistance (inferior to a Universal weight-stack and barbells), resistance is inadequately applied to muscles throughout the range of motion and any acquired skill does not transfer to other activities.

> **The value of exercise should be judged by the quality of resistance and the range of motion over which the resistance is effective. . . TRX training fails on both counts.**

The first time I tried the basic movements of TRX—instruction card in hand—there were several that proved too difficult to assume a starting position, let alone begin. I thought I lacked the strength but soon changed my mind. On the second and third attempts, without having gained strength from the initial failures, I did better. I lacked skill—a skill I considered non-essential.

If you want to learn a variety of useless skills that produce minimal strength gains, try TRX. Ironically, the colorful straps are often attached to equipment that would clearly provide superior results.

The TRX concept was designed and developed by a Navy Seal who failed to match Arthur Jones' one-and-only perfect score on the Navy entrance exam (*he was underage at the time*). And I'll add: If the Seals used the TRX exclusively, they wouldn't be in half the shape they are; and if they did not use the TRX at all, they wouldn't miss a thing. Simply put: There's a Seal out there with a pocketful of money.

Experts claim that a cross-trained athlete is a better athlete. Where's the research? From a skill perspective, the only way to improve in a sport is to practice the sport, not a dozen other activities. From a conditioning perspective, the condition gained by playing a sport may possess a degree of specificity, but if you participate in another activity that increases strength, cardiovascular capacity or flexibility, it may benefit the target activity. The stimulus provided and strength gained by TRX training is not likely to produce or transfer that benefit.

Pilates

One day a client I was stretching asked in reference to a poster on a nearby wall, "What's that Pilates?" (pronounced as "PIE Lates"). My explanation that day may prove as effective as the critique that follows because, other than a 20-minute demo, I have never done Pilates. But I've read and seen enough to know that I'm not interested. Hardcore? Close-minded? Perhaps. Here's an outsider's view:

The Good (and "the Claimed"):

1. Pilates addresses muscles that are unique to those worked in traditional exercise settings, with an emphasis on the "core."
2. To strengthen any muscle(s) of the body is a good thing.
3. Pilates emphasizes stretching and flexibility increase.
4. It highlights proper movement patterns (form).
5. Pilates believes that all of the energy for exercise is generated from the center of the body outward—a center referred to as the "powerhouse." A strong inner foundation forms the basis of general strength and movement.
6. Pilates demands concentration on every part of your body and specifically, on the parts creating the movement. Control is essential to performance.
7. Breathing in a specific pattern and with great depth is important for the delivery of oxygen to the working muscles.
8. Every movement has purpose and each is related to a greater whole.
9. Movement should be performed with fluidity.
10. The novelty and group aspects of Pilates attract people who might not otherwise perform exercise.

The Bad (a critique of "The Good and The Claimed," in order):

1. Strengthening "core" muscles is important only if you believe they are as important as Pilates enthusiasts make them out to be. I believe otherwise: Abdominal muscles take care of themselves by becoming indirectly involved in every physical effort. And while indirect does not trump direct, the core does not need to be reminded "to engage" before every repetition of exercise. It happens automatically and the constant prompt may become a distraction. The nervous system can only control so many muscles at once.

   The most important muscles of the core *cannot* be strengthened by Pilates exercise. One session on the MedX Lumbar Extension machine would do more to strengthen the muscles that extend the spine than months of Pilates training.

2. Where and when possible, muscles should be strengthened through a full range of motion. Mat Pilates (performed without equipment) features many static poses. Research demonstrates that in the majority of subjects, strength gain is limited to the angle(s) of work in both static and dynamic efforts (see Chapter 8). Full-range strength is impossible with static exercise. Pilates' machine exercises may provide a greater range of motion but I doubt a complete one.

Effective muscle-targeting occurs when the muscle is the prime mover, directly involved in—or the direct cause of—the motion. In most Pilates' movements the abdominals act as non-primary assistants. To what degree do they work and how much strength do they gain? The fact that a client can now perform a more challenging task or hold a position for a longer time is not an objective measure of an increase in strength, tissue architecture or force output. It may be a function of—as with TRX use—improved skill. But it sure puts a smile on faces.

The strength benefits of Pilates are limited by the absence of high levels of intensity. From what I've observed, exercise is not continued to a point of momentary muscle failure. When clients report how HARD it is, it is more likely related to the difficulty of learning a new skill—which is not a criticism of the professionals trying to provide their clients with a challenging workout.

The commercial claims that Pilates will leave you "refreshed, relaxed and rejuvenated" were never part of Jones' vocabulary. And the claim of a complete body transformation after thirty sessions could be expedited by the use of other forms of exercise that provide higher levels of intensity:

"This is not to suggest that some strengthening and conditioning does not take place, but that the extent to which this occurs is far

---

It is impossible to understand anything that you cannot measure; and thus it unavoidably follows that you cannot determine the results of any action until you can accurately measure any such results. Arthur Jones

more modest than the industry believes and with far better methods available to enhance an individual's physical function." [2]

The popularity of Pilates is due to aggressive marketing. The common claim that Pilates "creates long, lean" [3] muscles is attractive to those who despise the opposite, but nonetheless absurd. The length of a muscle is genetically predetermined and can only increase as a momentary adaptation to a movement. The same result can be achieved by full-range exercise on a machine or by targeted stretching movements.

3. The focus on good form during exercise is a must. However, the claim that proper movement patterns established during Pilates carries over to activities of daily living is a stretch. Skill does NOT transfer unless movements are IDENTICAL. In this case, they are not.

4. The "powerhouse" is powerful imagery but not true. Energy for exercise is generated by the muscle initiating the movement and not necessarily from the center of the body.

5. Concentration on muscles or body parts during exercise may promote good form by slowing speed of movement, but it adds little to the effort or result. If you can barely perform ten repetitions of an exercise, such focus is not likely to get you to eleven. The control element demanded of Pilates' movements extends to the realm of pointing toes, rotating wrists, positioning fingers and establishing a specific head position or degree of arch in the low back—all of which may appeal to the "grace" and "ballet" aspirations of the client but have little to do with physiological stimulation. Concentration on a perfect movement each time reflects the extent to which Pilates has become "skill" training.

6. Specific breathing patterns during exercise are not as important as projected. Your body will sense the required need and respond accordingly. Breathing does not increase results, but its lack may prevent them.

7. All exercise should have purpose and intent both at ground level and in the larger scheme of things. It may depend on your definition of exercise. I like this one:

   "Vigorous muscular activity, with the intent to cause inroads (loss) in functional ability, in order to stimulate physiological adaptive response, to increase, maintain, or slow the regression of said functional ability." [4]

   That doesn't sound like the Pilates I've seen.

8. While fluid movements promote better form and increase safety, increased function should be based on targeting muscles (through isolation) and building strength. Fluid movement is less functional than strength and does not transfer to activities of daily living as claimed.

9. Doing something is, in most cases, better than doing nothing—but the focus should remain on physiology, as Brenda Hutchins suggests in her critique, *"Pilates emphasizes the easy and fun social setting over the exercise requirement for control and hard work."* [5] In the early 1970's Brenda worked for Nautilus Sports/Medical Industries.

The claims made by Pilates organizations represent an attempt to prop-up what we commonly encounter in the fitness industry. There are better ways to use your time.

And The Ugly:

The contributions of Joseph Pilates and Arthur Jones to the field of exercise had little in common. They both shared a desire to "help" people through exercise—a notable endeavor—but that's where it ended. Pilates developed tools and a system that worked within the confines of the resistance available at the time—pulleys, springs, bodyweight, etc. Jones realized the limitations of the resistance and sought to change its application by working within the confines of muscle function. How can resistance be applied directly? How much resistance should be applied at this angle of movement? His work led to tools that better satisfied the needs of muscles and to a system that more aggressively met those needs. There can be little discussion about the comparative results in regard to the five potential benefits of exercise.

The pioneers compared favorably, however, in another realm.

While Joseph Pilates was still alive, two of his students opened facilities of their own. One, a hockey player named Bob Seed, opened a "Pilates" studio across town in New York City. To attract and satisfy his clients he opened earlier in the morning than his mentor, which didn't sit well. Joe showed up early one morning with a gun and ran Seed out of town.

Jones did not use a gun to etch or protect his niche in the marketplace but had it within reach for "if and when" necessary. At Arthur's funeral, son Gary quoted his dad: *"I've killed 650 elephants in my day, and 65 men. I rather regret the elephants."*

Kettlebell Workouts

Approximately ten years ago I returned to my place of birth, Welland, Ontario to see what remained of a once thriving steel town along the famous canal that linked Lake Erie to Lake Ontario. It wasn't much. The steel industry had folded, Canada's only John Deere® plant had left and all the downtown bridges that fascinated me as a boy were rendered dysfunctional, replaced by a wider canal that bypassed the city. The telephone directory led me to the only gym in town, the "Galaxy 2000" located in a two-story building formerly occupied by Switson Industries, a small-parts manufacturing firm in the heart of the industrial zone. It was there that I got my first glimpse of kettlebells.

A few steps up and right of the entrance foyer was a room of "museum quality" that housed as much rust as equipment. A row of high, shallow windows provided just enough light to reduce the chance of injury if you dared stay. The lower left corner of the room housed several handles that joined what looked like two cannonballs, and beside them, the kettlebells in loose array. They, too, looked liked cannonballs, each with its own handle. I expected legendary Canadian strong-man Louis Cyr to appear, but it didn't happen. Not much happened in that room.

Several years ago kettlebells resurfaced wrapped in colorful plastic and I had my first glimpse of their use—people swinging weights. And what I thought was "bad form" was "what they do" with kettlebells.

The handle is positioned beyond the weight's center of gravity which allows limbs to travel with less control through their range of motion. The momentum created can force limbs and muscles to exceed their safe range, which is why kettlebell trainers go to great lengths to establish a safe position from which to work. They must. And they go to great lengths to assure that range of motion is not exceeded—a practice that can lead to flexibility loss, as it does with cardiovascular exercise.

The claims made by kettlebell specialists are threefold: increased strength, power and cardiovascular condition. They are right on one but not on the others. Kettlebell training has the same potential as dumbbells to increase muscle strength but the way they are used makes that claim as murky as their 18th-century Russian origin. "Swinging weights" does NOT build strength as effectively as "lifting weights." Speed can destroy limbs and strength gains. And more: Demonstrating power in the gym has NOTHING to do with developing power or improving power on the field.

In a recent study at California State University, exercise physiologist Jared Coburn and his associates compared the effectiveness of kettlebell exercises to traditional weight-lifting exercises. Specifically, they compared the kettlebell swing, accelerated squat and "goblet" squat to the traditional high dead-lift, power clean and back squat. Following six weeks of training with thirty untrained subjects, they measured strength and power. Both groups improved. Gains were similar in measures of power (the vertical jump) but different in regard to strength: The barbell group increased by 13.6 percent, the kettlebell group by 4.5 percent. The difference was attributed to the increased momentum with kettlebells.

An aside: *The strength increase recorded by both groups is pitiful compared to that produced by Project Total Conditioning, where the implementation of superior tools, proper supervision, high levels of intensity and better form proved that strength and power can be obtained through the use of slow, controlled movements.*

Kettlebell training was recently defined by a Toronto newspaper and praised for its simplicity and cardiovascular benefits: *"A few basic movements with a single piece of equipment can raise heart rate and recruit muscles throughout the body, in contrast to traditional weight training, which uses specific exercises to isolate individual muscles."* [6] The use of many muscles at once makes kettlebell training cardiovascular—but how much so?

Research scientists at Truman State University in Missouri compared a ten-minute kettlebell swing routine (thirty-five seconds of swinging, alternated with twenty-five seconds of rest) to a ten-minute treadmill run. They kept the effort as constant as they could by matching the "perceived effort" of the two activities, specifically adjusting the speed of the treadmill to match the effort perceived by the kettlebell workout. The kettlebell routine maintained heart rates above 85 percent of maximum, enough for an "effect." And despite the fact that subjects had to continually increase the speed of the treadmill to keep up with the effort level of the kettlebell workout, the treadmill work burned more calories and consumed more oxygen (25% versus 39%). The conclusion of the study was that the aerobic effect of kettlebell training was "decent" but did not stack up to traditional training. And there's more . . .

In a University of Waterloo study (Waterloo, Ontario), Stuart McGill reported that kettlebell training exposed spinal vertebrae to more lateral than compression force. Lateral force puts vertebral facets at risk, especially as rotational movement reaches the limits of its range. Once again, how you perform an exercise is more important than what the resistance weighs or what tool you use.

If strength is the most important reason to perform exercise in the first place, you might reconsider kettlebells.

Vibration Training

In the late 1960's the Olympic Games were inundated by athletes from the European communist bloc hell-bent on showing the world the superiority of their system—and they did. Their dominance was rumored to include the identification of talent at an early age, the development of that talent through elite training schools and, most important, the use of steroids. The chemical warfare was masked by claims of secret strength-training methods and technology, some of which were reported in Joe Weider's magazines throughout that era.

Vibration training evolved from the space program in the former Soviet Union—an attempt to expose astronauts to gravitational force (and ultimately, some exercise) in space. Its theory evolves from the formula: **Force = Mass x Acceleration**. Muscles produce force. Stronger muscles produce greater force. Therefore, anything that increases the force a muscle *can* produce is a plus. Traditional strength training increases the mass (the amount of weight) to augment force output; vibration training affects the acceleration component by increasing the earth's gravitational pull (from 1.0 G to as much as 1.8 G's). This increases the force requirement and fiber recruitment of muscles, which accelerates and magnifies strength gains. So they claim.

There is no research that directly compares resistance training to vibration training, although some studies compare training done with and without vibration. In a recent research review, the cited studies demonstrated no significant difference in strength gains between performing exercise with or without vibration: research on squats (2004, 2009; by *B. Ronnestad*); research on dynamic biceps curls (2007) and knee extensions (2008; by *K. Moran and J. Luo*); and a review of literature (2007; by *Nordlund and Thorstensson*). *"The research to date,"* the review concluded, *"appears not to support the use of VT (vibration training) for improving strength to a greater extent than resistance training alone."* [7]

The potential for vibration in strength training may not be as rosy as painted. Some reviews warn of "the physiological hazards associated with exposure to vibration" and certification programs shy away from contraindications. Some trainees experience headaches; others can't tolerate the sensation. Vibration involves impact, and impact—I was taught—is negative. When all cards are on the table, I wouldn't be surprised to see vibration training categorized with plyometrics or dynamic muscle testing: "Danger to no purpose."

At first glance vibration training looks like nothing more than a flurry of bodyweight exercises on a vibrating platform. It can, however, be performed using barbells or other forms of resistance but most trainers choose not to, for reasons: The additional gravity encountered during vibration on a platform *supposedly* provides the added resistance needed to stimulate change; and the *claimed* increase in recovery-time required after vibration exercise makes trainers tentative. Since nothing can be measured or compared, no one really knows what happens. Convenient.

The self-proclaimed leader in vibration technology, Power Plate©, has chords that protrude from the sides of its platform to add exercise variety. The vibration transmitted via these chords, however, is so muted that the manufacturer suggests two options to improve quality: One, the chord can be adjusted to a position that creates more friction as it exits the machine; and two, it can be pulled faster which increases friction and provides the "feel" of greater resistance. When I heard the second suggestion (from a Master trainer), a familiar alarm rang in my head: *"The next time somebody suggests that you move suddenly during any form of either exercise or testing,"* said Arthur Jones, *"smile and walk away, because you are talking to a fool."* More than the tool should be questioned when the manufacturer recommends bad form to improve its function and results. In either case, the increase in resistance provided by the chords working *at their best* is inadequate for someone who requires hard work.

Vibration websites reference more than 180 studies that demonstrate the positive effect of their product on a multitude of training variables beyond strength: power production, recovery, flexibility, body composition, cellulite reduction, local muscular and cardiovascular endurance, health and wellness parameters, balance, bone density, circulation, etc.—leaving the impression that vibration *may have been the missing link* in Western-performance training in the 1960's. It was not.

Some claims are substantiated. The Power Plate is effective for flexibility. Vibration restrains sensors that inhibit muscles from reaching length limits, thereby allowing more stretch. Cardiovascular claims are also valid if exercise is performed sequentially with limited rest between efforts—a method that produces a cardiovascular benefit with *any* form of exercise.

Some claims are unsubstantiated. Bone density allegations are poor because strength gains are poor. The Power Plate flagship study (published in *The Journal of Bone and Mineral Research,* 2004) boasts a 1.5% increase in "bone density" over a twenty-four-week training period. According to Margaret Martin, PT, a therapist who reviewed the study, *"The reason the Power Plate group showed an increase in hip area bone density over the study period—compared to the other groups—was not due to the benefits of the PPVP (Power Plate Vibration Platform). It was a result of the exercise program that they followed."* The Power Plate group performed progressive weight-bearing exercises, while the traditional-trained group performed non-weight-bearing endurance exercises that were not progressive—and have yet to demonstrate a positive effect on bone density.

In any case, the 1.5% increase is dismal. Many studies (Pollock, 1992; Menkes, 1993; Braith and others, 1996) demonstrate greater increases using traditional strength-training methods and equipment.

Other claims (from the Power Plate website) are absurd:

- *"As it turns out, couples that exercise together strengthen more than their muscles—they also strengthen their romantic connection."*
- The mention of cellulite reduction evokes memories of the European approach around 1950. Cellulite is not a *special* fat that requires *special* treatment.
- *"Acceleration training on a Power Plate stimulates fast-twitch muscle fibers and athletes who use Power Plate machines over time experience a dramatic increase in explosive strength, motor learning, muscular endurance and overall agility."* Hardly. Fast-twitch fibers are activated by intensity, not vibration or speed of movement. Explosive training is flat-out dangerous. Motor learning cannot increase on a Power Plate because of the laws governing specificity and transfer. Local muscular endurance and strength are one and the same. Agility is genetically fixed and not subject to change.

. . . what next?

The theory behind vibration raises more questions. The corporal instability created by whole-body vibration is addressed by muscle recruitment to restore stability. When muscle contracts, blood is directed towards the need which amplifies the importance of relaxing *non-working* muscles. There is no choice with vibration training. Full-body vibration directs circulation to the whole body which may justify the claims of greater muscle recruitment and potential for strength gain. But the circulatory mechanism is a closed-hydraulic system with a limited supply. Why involve all muscles when your target is only one or two?

If vibration training works as claimed, why not apply it to exercises with superior resistance? Vibrate a Nautilus machine or an entire gym floor. In this field—ridiculous is often just around the corner.

Arthur Jones applauded any innovation that made exercise harder and more productive. *"Design it, build it, strap it on your back and head off down the runway,"* he said, *"then it will either fly or it won't; but until you try it, you will never know for sure."*

I don't think vibration will fly.

Conclusion

I worked during four summers to get myself through college. For three, I was employed by Ford Motor Company®—worked in their glass manufacturing plant in Niagara Falls, Ontario. One summer they were slow to hire so I picked up a job at the Page-Hershey plant in Welland. Page-Hershey manufactured large metal tubes (aqueducts) that served the transportation and construction industries. By comparison the place was filthy, noisy and dangerous. One day, the foreman paired me with an Italian man who had worked there most of his life. Luigi and I worked side by side for a couple of hours, each wearing a pair of safety glasses, heavy-duty ear protectors and a hard-hat. At break we removed our head gear and dashed to the quieter confines of the lunch room. Luigi spoke first.

"Hey, boy," he asked. "Whatsa you name?"

"Gary," I replied.

"Oh," he said with a pleasant smile, "Jeddy."

"No, Gary," I repeated with increased clarity.

"OK, Jeddy," he insisted. "Coma down here, Jeddy. We clean 'em up a lilla bit."

That wasn't the end of it. When I jokingly told my high-school buddies, they began calling me "Jeddy"—and the name stuck.

Luigi had good intentions and listened closely, but couldn't quite get it right. He couldn't wrap his tongue around the hard "G."

Sad to say, the Page-Hershey was eerily similar to my ultimate field of choice—exercise. When I first entered, there was a lot of noise—not the same kind, but of a similar magnitude. Everyone was busy doing their thing. It was deafening and from all directions, but you got used to it. There was always someone to show you the ropes and you didn't challenge things. Luigi knew. He said to me at lunch one day, "Company try to screw us, Jeddy." If they were, he still showed day after day and left his challenge in the lunch room, all forty years of it.

In my field, trainer certification groups and entrepreneurs rule the roost. They dictate the tone, direct the conversation and provide the noise. We show up day after day and, with alarming frequency, stumble across "something new"—a gadget, a program, a theory. Sometimes we chew it over in the lunch room with rarely a challenge. The "something new" cost "X" dollars and is here to stay. So, we don our head gear and deal with it—and the pile grows. Whether the new requires ear protectors, hard hats or both, most of it's not worth the paper it's written on. But its creators know full-well that the longer it lingers, the greater the chance it sticks.

Trainers and trainees have been so inundated with noise that we are often forced to wade through an ocean to wrap a tongue around what fact remains. The word "NO" has no hard "G." What the field needs is a *lilla* backbone to prevent it from going the way of the Page-Hershey—down the tubes.

REFERENCES

[1] Fisher, J., Steele, J., Bruce-Low, S., Smith, D., "Evidence-Based Resistance Training Recommendations," *Medicina Sportiva*, 15 (3): 147-162, 2011.

[2] www.mindfullmoves.com.

[3] Morrison, R., "Pilates: The Irrefutable Truth," *Synergy 2007*.

[4] Johnston, B.D, *Fitness Analytics*: Book II, 607, 1995-2007

[5] Hutchins, B., "Why Not Pilates?" www.renaissanceexercise.com.

[6] Hutchinson, A., *The Globe and Mail*, June 10, 2012.

[7] Fisher, J., Steele, J., Bruce-Low, S., Smith, D., "Evidence-Based Resistance Training Recommendations," *Medicina Sportiva*, 15 (3): 147-162, 2011.

PART III

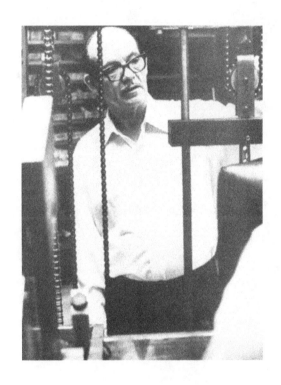

Beyond The Bamboozle

CHAPTER 20

··

Proper Strength Training
And Beyond

**Fifty years ago, most of the commonly accepted
theories in this field were wrong; today almost all of
these same myths are still widely accepted, and in the
meantime, hundreds of other superstitions have taken
root. So we are now stuck with most of the old myths
and a lot of new ones.**

Arthur Jones

I rarely think of tomorrow, let alone the future . . . but I met someone
who did. I attended the University of North Carolina at Greensboro
for post-graduate work in 1972 and, coming from Canada, knew
nothing about the place. I soon discovered that the school had converted
from "female" to "co-ed" the year before which made it tough to eat in the
cafeteria the first few weeks. During one lunch I stumbled through a bevy of
"Belles" and bee-lined to a sparse corner when I heard a pleasant, *"Won't
you join us?"* To my right was a young lady wearing a colorful head scarf
and round, thick eyeglasses. She was flanked by two strange men. Twenty
minutes of Southern hospitality I thought—what the heck. They wrapped up
introductions before I could land: Consuela, Dick and Davey. And before
I could locate my napkin, I was confronted by the dreaded, *"What's your
sign?"* My reply ruined the meal, *"Pisces."* As I reached for a fork, Consuela
intercepted my hand and started reading my palm. Lunch became a hybrid
of pain and humor—enough of the latter to introduce my roommate to the
trio the next time we saw them. Sure enough, within seconds, Consuela

had his hand, palm up. From that day on, knowing that our futures were of limited significance, we opted for "the late shift" or simply waved to the lady with the colorful head scarf from the far side of the room. She was hard to miss, but we managed.

Since then, I've not been back—too many lines on my palms to keep it brief and afraid that history will repeat. History has that habit whether we learn from it or not—and most times we don't. With that in mind and no time-frame—and with all due respect to Consuela—I look into a palm that has performed more than its fair share of exercise and tell you what I see.

The future of exercise lies in two directions:

- The field must first define its product(s).
- Word must then reach the medical community.

The parameters of cardiovascular training are well defined. We know what heart-rate zones provide exercise and what represents too little or too much. Parameters have also been established for those with heart conditions. And, other than defining the most effective way to stimulate cardiovascular change, little controversy has occurred along the way.

In contrast, progressive resistance training remains undefined—confusion, opinion, myth and lies—no one knows where to turn. The sad part: It is—by far—the most important product the field has to offer. Muscle strength is the window to athletic performance, to mobility, corporal reconstruction, injury prevention, cardiovascular fitness and to flexibility. Strength is the gateway to *every* potential benefit of exercise. Cardiovascular exercise is the gateway to the heart alone—a message that is rarely exposed.

And it may not matter: Those on the receiving end are few and far between. Few people perform exercise because they are inherently lazy (human nature) and their time is occupied by an increasing number of distractions that are *not* physical. The fitness industry has survived by luring the public with fun things, things they can do, easy choices—whatever it takes. The success has been financial at times, but rarely physiological. The long-term effect of *"doing something is better than doing nothing"* can only lead to failure. The few that are attracted to exercise see so little gain with "the easier choices" that they quit. Can you blame them? A huge effort for most with little to no reward—I'd quit too. Exercise must be hard enough to stimulate change that can be appreciated.

The personal-training side of the industry has provided little assistance. Many trainers are so busy running about collecting certifications that they are utterly confused. Each national group has an agenda that vies for power on the big scene. How many trainers can we sign up? How many conferences can we host? It's all about quantity, not quality; about brainwashing, not education. The poor guy at the end of the stick—the one you ask for advice—doesn't know where to turn. Certification organizations, intentions aside, have done more harm than good—only added to the pile—and as long as trainers send in their dues, there's no end in sight. Exercise education should revert to a four-year process with a curriculum based on truth, not interpretation. There's enough information out there to reach a consensus on resistance training but it may never be done.

If trainers ever get off the toilet and they might somewhere down the line, they will come to realize:

- Strength training is more important than cardiovascular training.
- Stronger muscles are the key to increased function.
- The strengthening process should proceed *without* concern for the ultimate goal.
- Muscles generate, register and absorb force. That's it. The nervous system determines the functional puzzle.
- The best way to strengthen muscles is through the application of isolated, direct, high-intensity, full-range exercise—the dosage determined by accurate testing.

The medical equivalent of *"What's your sign?"* is the dreaded, *"What should I do about my condition, Doctor?"* Many physicians understand the role of exercise in solving the problem but are just as likely to say, *"Pisces."* Perhaps they don't know, or are not expected to know specifics. But as professionals they're expected to reply—which is often weak or misinformed, again, despite intentions. The uninformed provide the standard, *"Walk or swim"*—cardiovascular choices that, to date, pose no threat to life. The informed are forced to draw from a well of information that's all over the map. Some of the worst form I've seen in gyms belongs to doctors who either know nothing about strength training or take advice from muscle-heads who aren't even literate.

Until the field of exercise defines what is true and what is not, it will never have the impact that it could. The tools are there and many questions have already been answered by logic, physics and research—but the stumbling blocks of ego, money and fraud remain.

Physicians loom large in the success of the endeavor. For the most part the public has little faith in the exercise community: Ask twenty trainers or national organizations and you get twenty opinions. But the public *has* faith in the medical community. When John Doe finally obtains accurate information from a physician who has access to the accurate information he or she seeks, the ball will begin to roll.

The fitness industry might do better to borrow a page from Arthur Jones, "*. . . the minimum amount of exercise that will produce the desired result. Anything in excess of that minimum is by definition unnecessary, therefore illogical . . . and possibly contra-productive.*" It doesn't take much proper exercise to produce the desired result—and should take *less* in the future.

Equipment

Cardiovascular equipment currently provides users with all the information needed to produce, monitor and record results. Strength-training tools provide nothing. The guidelines required to successfully use an exercise machine are derived from research and trial and error, and measured by testing tools that are inadequate for the purpose. That must change.

Arthur Jones initiated the development of valid strength-testing machines in the early 1970's and, a decade later, challenged the technology standard in the medical field—isokinetics—by building a "super" isokinetic machine

---

Until the field of exercise defines what is true and what is not, it will never have the impact that it could.

to expose its shortcomings. In the process he identified the ingredients of proper testing and developed safe, accurate tools to measure isolated muscle function. Some listened. Twenty years of dynamic testing soon disappeared and the information gleaned from a proper evaluation was incorporated into the design of exercise protocols that met the exact needs of a muscle.

Jones developed five such rehabilitative machines that featured isolated muscle testing in a static mode and full-range exercise in a dynamic mode. And he hinted that not all muscles can be isolated—but there are more than five. With his blueprint it wouldn't take much to develop a more extensive and affordable set of testing/exercise tools to increase the flow of information between testing and training centers—information that accurately defines the characteristics and needs of every major muscle group so that everyone knows *exactly* how to proceed.

So much for testing: How about exercise? In the late 1970's Jones published an article entitled, "The Future of Exercise—An Opinion." He described a form of exercise he called "infimetric" that involved lifting with one limb while resisting with the other. That is, while one arm (or leg) pushed against a pad or movement arm, the effort was resisted by the other limb pulling in the opposite direction. Since muscles were stronger lowering than lifting *under all circumstances*, the working muscle would *always* confront an unlimited source of resistance—hence the name. The infimetric tools had no external weight stack, low friction and connected to a computer that provided instant information to the trainee concerning form and intensity. It recorded the information and automatically adjusted the program to meet the needs of the next session. By the early 1980's Jones had developed a complete line of "infimetric" tools but that's as far as it got. He abandoned the project because, I assume, he couldn't solve all of the problems, which may have left it ripe for some other genius.

Future testing tools *must* meet the requirements of safety and accuracy; future exercise equipment *must* provide full-range exercise. The immediate future appears dim for the latter.

Months ago a committee consisting of clients and staff from our fitness-and-wellness center in Florida ventured to neighboring facilities to gather information related to the purchase of equipment for a "new" center.

Following a hands-on tour of Cybex® machines at one site, I asked the salesman why the leading manufacturers have not adopted the MedX® system of lifting weight stacks. MedX machines lever weights from the bottom which eliminates 90% of the friction that exists in the old double guide-rod system. His answer was blunt: *"There's no demand in the marketplace."*

". . . for quality?"

"No," he replied, *"No demand for machines."*

For decades, impressive rows of exercise machines provided a stimulus to attract people to gyms and the structure that many clients sought. Their efficiency and effectiveness helped retain the attraction. The current trend to functional training has no use for machines and that has made an impression on gym floors. New facilities appear empty—and empty requires supervision and ultimately greater cost.

On a larger scale, the persistent attacks on the threat posed by Nautilus machines in the 1970's have come to fruition. The public wants something new, something that makes exercise interesting and time pass more quickly. The trend does *not* signal the demise of machines but injects a bump along the road of history—and history repeats:

The first "big" development in the field of exercise involved the introduction of individual machines ("medical gymnastics") in 1857 by Dr. Gustaf Zander at the Medico-Mechanical Institute in Stockholm, Sweden. There, he developed forty different exercise machines activated by muscular action or driven by steam, gas or electric power. According to Arthur Jones, *"He (Zander) was clearly aware of, and obviously understood, many of the actual requirements for proper exercise that I introduced in early Nautilus machines."* Jones would have saved a lot of time had he known of Zander's work (an attempt to vary resistance during exercise to meet the calculated requirements of muscles through a full range of motion). Zander's machines were still in use in major hospitals 100 years later.

The next "big" development was the introduction of barbells in 1902—resistance with a handle. Then came the Universal® machine of the

1960's, mere copies of free-weight exercises with the same problems and deficiencies. The not-so-big step is where the field has retreated today.

The next advance was "the thinking man's barbell"—the Nautilus® machine. What Zander missed, Jones did not, and the field is still trying to figure it out.

Case in point: Friction affects the function and longevity of all exercise machines. Yet, when our search committee visited one facility, I was astonished that their new LifeFitness® machines had a side weight stack with its own pair of guide-rods. Two for the main weight stack, two for the auxiliary—double the friction every time you add five pounds. No wonder there's no demand.

Negative-work Potential

The next significant discovery in exercise will tap the muscle's potential for lowering weight. In the early 1980's I entered a gym in Miami, Florida with world champion water-skier, Ana Maria Carrasco. My mission was to salvage a routine from a set of old Nautilus machines. When we finished, Ana and I wandered over to a handful of computerized LifeFitness® machines that had attracted a crowd. The new tools felt "normal" during the lifting phase but added 40% to the resistance during the lowering phase. The idea was brilliant but the execution was not. The transition from lifting to lowering exposed the muscles to a dramatic jolt. No wonder there's no demand.

Another attempt was recently made in Stockholm, Sweden by a man with a different approach. Mats Thulin developed a weight stack that assumed a 45-degree tilt as it lifted and an upright position as it lowered. The hydraulic transition reduced the resistance by 29% during the lift but applied the full value during the lowering phase, making exercise feel *equally* hard on the up and the down. Ellington Darden visited the "X-Force®" facility in 2008 and, during one exercise, reached an ideal inroad of 21% in forty-two seconds as opposed to sixty seconds on an equivalent traditional machine. The harder work required during the lowering phase reduced his training time by 30% and he and his host finished a complete eight-exercise whole-body workout in less than fifteen minutes. On the downside, the machines debuted in 2011 to complaints of expense, the potential for mechanical difficulties and "a poor cam on the leg-extension machine."

When someone gets it right, it will decrease workout time and frequency—and change exercise forever.

The Training System

If and when the field of exercise seeks and discovers the unbiased truth, two facts will emerge:

- **Strength will jump to the forefront of training.**
- **The method to acquire strength will be *"the minimum amount to produce the desired result."* It will be brief, hard and infrequent.**

The only thing not likely to change—and a major stumbling block—is human nature. "More is better" with most, and exercise is no exception.

Another stumbling block is the industry itself. It cares more about survival than truth and has spent a great deal of energy catering to special interest groups: Athletes because of their influence and "perceived" special needs, and women because they are the industry's major consumers.

Since the arrival of something other than barbells, the field of exercise has recognized the potential of female participation. As a result they inundated the market with ideas that attracted women—group classes, Yoga, Pilates, Swiss balls, latex bands and gadgets—things that minimize strength and maximize rhetoric. In my opinion, women have missed a lot—including the truth.

At the other end, the athlete's constant search for a competitive edge has driven the fitness industry to discover something beyond just "lifting weights," which results in the following:

1. It makes athletes feel special because they are training specifically for the needs of their activity.

2. It makes them believe that how they currently prepare forms an integral part of their success.
3. It influences the next generation who are motivated to train like their heroes.
4. . . . and it makes the pile higher.

The truth is:

1. Athletes are special people but do NOT require special training (as far as strength is concerned).
2. Most athletes have tried so many things over their careers that they don't know what worked and what didn't . . .
3. . . . but they invariably think they do. More often than not, their training has held them back and led the field of exercise down a path that defies logic, research and common sense.
4. The pile has grown.

On a recent visit to Canada, I spent an afternoon with a friend in Stoney Creek, Ontario—near where I attended university. John Turner, an Arthur Jones fan, has a high-intensity web-site, lectures around the country and is humored by the way athletes train. With the 2012 Olympics in London on deck the national networks featured a number of profiles on the preparation of Canada's hopefuls—similar to what I had witnessed in the United States. The chains, ropes, plyometric activities and explosive weight-training—generally non-productive and dangerous things performed on lousy equipment—led John to ask, *"Does the Olympic Committee need a loan?"*

DNA makes—by far—the dominant contribution to athletic success and training makes a *weak* claim for second. If U.S. athletes are so successful *because* of their training, why are Canada's athletes so unsuccessful doing the same? When the world wakes up to the importance of strength and emphasizes a rational way to get there, then you'll see *real* performance. As Jones suggested, *"A stronger athlete is a better athlete."* With trends as they are, today's athletes are not as strong as they could or should be—*because* of their training. The human body is capable of incredible things if human nature and the field of exercise get out of its way.

The future will eventually focus, as it must, on the development of strength through proper training. Then, and only then, will all of the potential benefits fall into place . . . and the field of exercise take a long-awaited step in the direction of "truth."

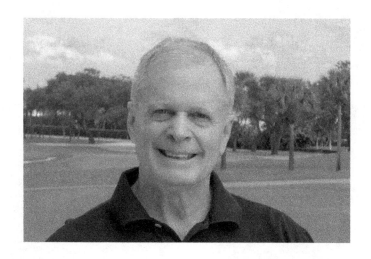

Gary Bannister received Bachelor's degrees in English and Physical Education from McMaster University in Hamilton, Ontario, and a Master's Degree in Physical Education from the University of North Carolina at Greensboro. He coached golf, soccer and basketball four years at Averett College in Danville, Virginia, and taught four years at Colegio Internacional de Caracas (an American high school in Venezuela). In 1980, he opened the first Nautilus gym and, eight years later, the first MedX rehabilitation center in South America. Since returning to the United States in 1990, he has worked in fitness and rehabilitation centers as a certified trainer and MedX technician. In 2005 he published his first book, *In Arthur's Shadow*—a tribute to Nautilus/MedX inventor, Arthur Jones.